PD You and Me

Pauline Braathen
&
Ken O'Bryan

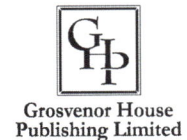

Grosvenor House
Publishing Limited

All rights reserved
Copyright © Pauline Braathen and Ken O'Bryan, 2014

The right of Pauline Braathen and Ken O'Bryan to be identified as the author of this work has been asserted by them in accordance with Section 78 of the Copyright, Designs and Patents Act 1988

The book cover picture is copyright to Pauline Braathen and Ken O'Bryan

This book is published by
Grosvenor House Publishing Ltd
28-30 High Street, Guildford, Surrey, GU1 3EL.
www.grosvenorhousepublishing.co.uk

This book is sold subject to the conditions that it shall not, by way of trade or otherwise, be lent, resold, hired out or otherwise circulated without the author's or publisher's prior consent in any form of binding or cover other than that in which it is published and
without a similar condition including this condition being imposed on the subsequent purchaser.

A CIP record for this book
is available from the British Library

ISBN 978-1-78148-741-9

Concept Pauline Mary Braathen

Text Ken O'Bryan PhD

Editor Sharon Clark

Design Andy Reilly

Copyright 2014...All Rights Reserved. No part of this work covered by the copyrights hereon may be reproduced or used in any form or by any means - graphic, electronic or mechanical, including photocopying, recording, taping, or information storage and retrieval systems without the prior written permission of the publisher.

PD
You and Me

Understanding and Challenging
Parkinson's Disease

This is the story of Pauline Braathen who has Parkinson's Disease

It is a positive and easy to read personal account of the symptoms, treatments and progress of PD

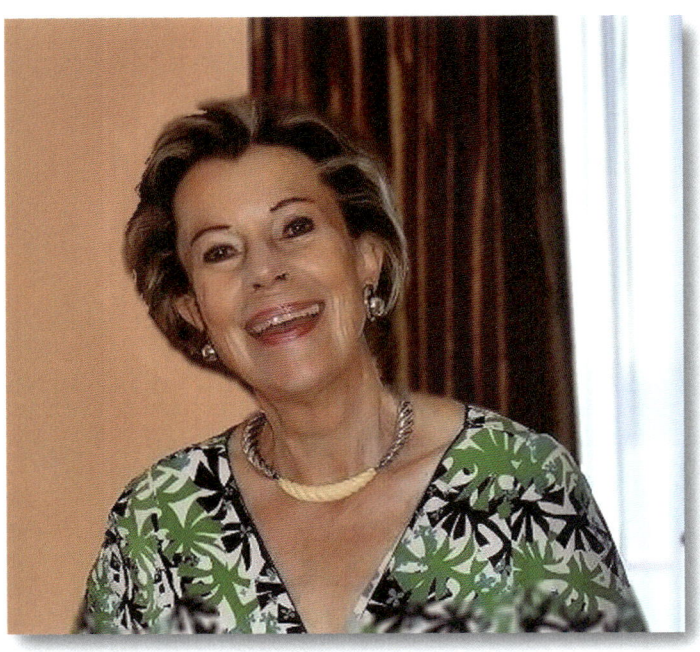

This is Pauline.

This is the story of her life with PD.

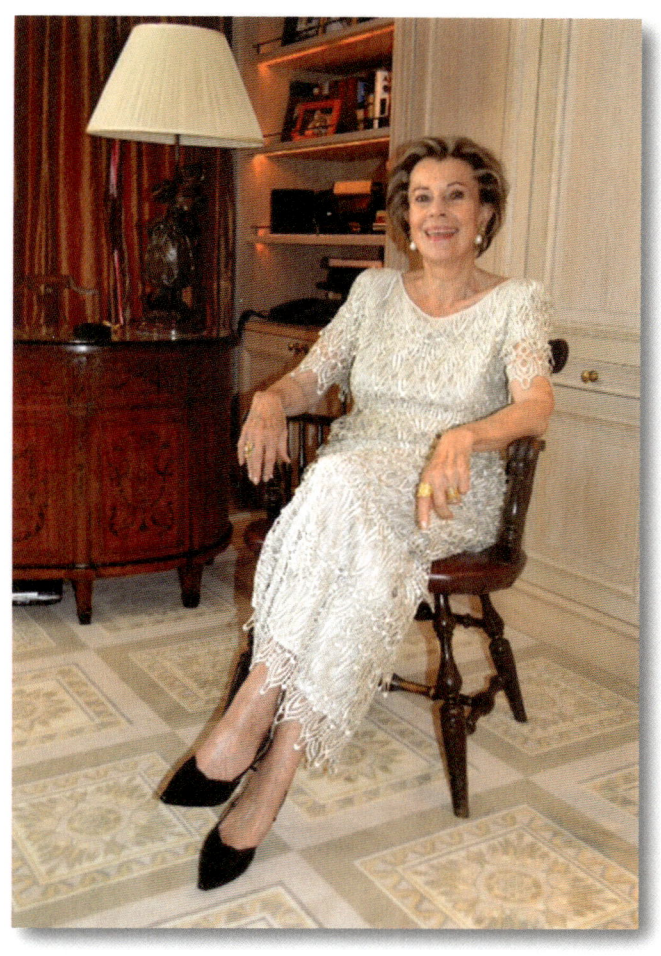

Being diagnosed with Parkinson's Disease is a serious matter.

But it is not the end of the world and it will be the start of a new experience in life that you can manage and control.

FEELING STRANGE – FEARING THE UNKNOWN

For quite a while now you have been worried.

Things are not like they used to be.

The hands that could tackle the finest of tools from tiny pliers to knitting needles have developed a tremor that seems to come from nowhere and then disappear – even when they are doing nothing.

Easy tasks that use small movements are somehow more difficult, slow and even impossible for a time.

You have noticed a stoop in your posture that was not there before. Climbing the stairs is strangely difficult. Walking in a straight line is not simple. Crossing a patch of rough pavement is tougher than it should be.

Turning in bed has become a little painful and your shoulder is stiff and sore.

One side of your body feels numb at times. One of your legs wants to quit helping to walk and sometimes needs dragging along.

And your kids complain that they can't read your handwriting anymore, so they buy you a laptop!

Eventually you go to the doctor. He asks a lot of questions, carries out some tests and tells you to come back later.

So you come back.

He asks you to sit down. Not a good beginning, you think!

Then he tells you the results. …………………………..

The diagnosis is **Parkinson's Disease**!

Well, you have heard of Parkinson's Disease, which we will call PD from now on.

But what is it, how is it treated, how long do you have, is there any hope? And a thousand more questions begin to come into your mind.

This is scary stuff!

The bad news about a diagnosis of PD is that you have it.

The good news is that an early diagnosis can greatly help in managing it, delaying it, and getting the most out of the very long time it takes PD to become worse.

And there is more good news!

It is not cancer and it won't kill you in a month or six months or two years. Something else is likely to get you long before PD will, if it ever does!

You are not suffering from Alzheimer's. Don't forget that!

Mad Cow Disease has been ruled out and unless you have enjoyed some long and losing boxing matches you have not got Boxer's Parkinsonism.

You do not have Multiple Sclerosis, a deadly stroke, or the Dreaded Lurgi or anything else that actually may be more noxious and immediate than PD.

Your heart is strong, blood pressure OK and most of you is functioning very well indeed.

PD is not yet advanced, or, at worst, it is in its middle stages of development.

But you do have PD and there it is. It is not going to go away.

Not yet anyway.

Still, who knows what the researchers will find anytime soon, and maybe there will be a real cure for it one day. Certainly there is an enormous effort being made worldwide at every level – diagnosis, assessment, treatment, a cure, and eventually prevention.

In the meantime you have a life to live and it can be positive, happy, fruitful, and long - or it can be scary, miserable, depressing, and still long.

So what are your options? Who can help you and how?

Your absolutely best resource is yourself. You hold the key to handling PD, living a good life in spite of it, taking control, making it work for every inch of progress along the way.

So this is where we start a reality program, based on an actual PD diagnosis and how one woman is dealing with it.

Pauline has been there and is here!

She has PD but she meets the disease head on and with verve, humor, determination, and real success. She has advice and support for all.

PD itself is no laughing matter, but you will find, just as Pauline has, that a sense of humor is a great help in dealing with it, even if that humor is occasionally just a little hard to find, or even a touch black!

KNOW YOUR ENEMY

Understanding Parkinson's Disease

Your own brain is the problem. But do not be too hard on it as it is also a big part of the solution.

PD affects you because of the lack of a key chemical that has slowly begun to be reduced in the brain. Unless treated, the chemical will continue to disappear and the condition will get steadily more difficult to deal with.

This chemical is called dopamine and a lot is known about it and how it works. In fact the solution to the dopamine problem may hold the key to an eventual understanding of the cause, the cure and the prevention of PD.

Getting the dopamine level in your brain to increase is a very important means of slowing the development of PD and reducing its symptoms.

So here is what you can think about, understand, and do to make your life as safe, full and rich as it can be, while we all wait for the scientists to beat PD once and for all.

One day they will and you want to be around to cheer them for it.

But they are not there yet.

In the meantime here is what to expect and how to handle it as the years go by. These are your options, choices, activities and likely outcomes.

YOU VERSUS PD – THE EARLY STAGES

OK. You have recovered from the shock of the diagnosis and you have started to ask the real questions.

Now you know you do not need to plan the succession, re-write your will, contact the distant family members, pay your gambling debts, or prepare for anything except the treatment of PD and the life you want to live.

You have time and lots of it. It may take more than 5-10 years for the tremors to get seriously worse, or for balance to get more difficult. And if the options you choose work as they can, then it will take much longer.

PD is the tortoise in this race but, like the other tortoise, it might eventually win unless it is delayed in every possible way.

So let's look at what can be done for you and what you can do for yourself.

There are at least 3 options so let's look at each of them.

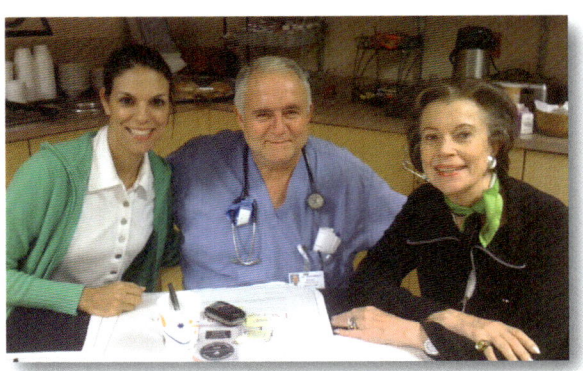

The three key elements in dealing with PD.
The doctor, the physiotherapist and most of all – You.

The Medical Options

The doctors will give you some good advice depending on how they see and assess you – which is not necessarily how you see yourself.

They will consider your age, working or retired, the stage of the PD progression, whether there is memory loss or confusion or other medical conditions that may affect treatment.

Doctors are not divinities!

Like anyone south of Heaven they can be and sometimes are wrong. They do their best, they offer alternatives and they should let you know the upside and downside of every treatment option.

Ask questions, get answers.

Look for a specialist, a neurologist, that you feel comfortable with for an ongoing professional relationship.

Know as much as you can about what is being suggested and how it is supposed to work, and especially what other effects, good and bad it can have. If you cannot do this for any reason get someone who can and will do it for you and with you.

Take control, listen, evaluate, and decide – it is your life and your choices.

The doctors will almost certainly look at the medication option first.

So we will too.

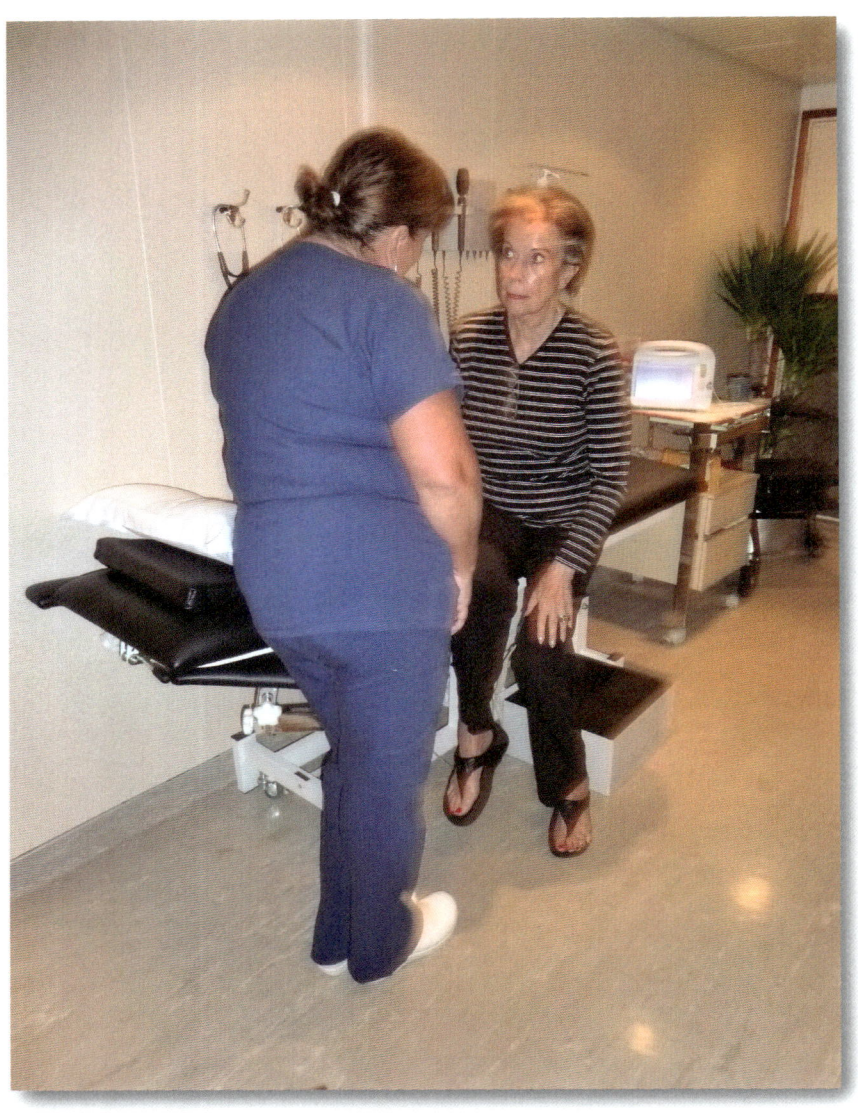

*This is the serious stuff. Listen well, ask questions, be informed.
You are the key person in it all - and you have the right to know.*

You already know by now that dopamine deficiency is at the centre of the problem. So the obvious answer seems to be to replace the dopamine and problem solved. The symptoms go away and PD is put on indefinite hold.

Nice idea, but not so easy.

Dopamine as such is not available as an injection or as a medicine. It has to be produced by the brain from some other substance. One of these is a registered medicine called Sinemet or a combination of levodopa and carbidopa. Where do they get these names!

Mainly from Latin, actually.

The funny thing is that the drug companies use a language that is officially dead to name their drugs to keep us alive! And some, such as Sinemet, are rather funny in themselves.

Sin does not mean being naughty. In Latin it means "without". And in the old Roman days an eating orgy was never complete without an emesis – or a comprehensive vomiting session.

So Sinemet means "without vomiting"!

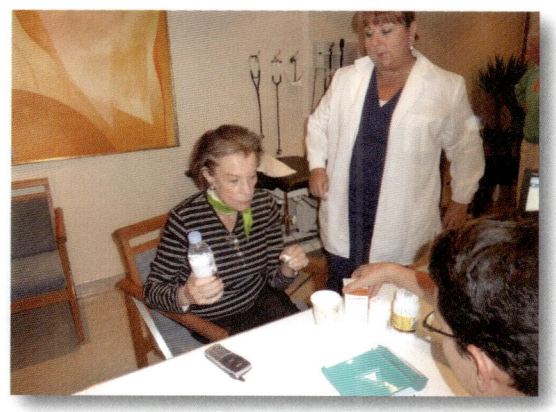

Not the happy hour!

Pauline started on Sinemet but her doctor changed her medication to Stalevo. It also contains carbidopa and levidopa with entacapone added to improve the effectiveness.

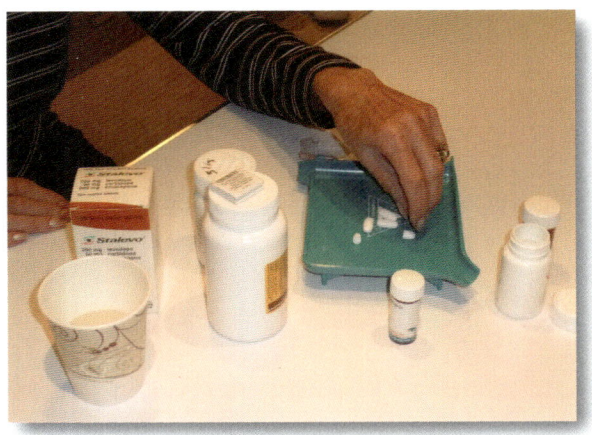

Don't mix these with that other sort of cocktail!

The PD treatment least liked by most is the medicine regime. But stick with it always. It will help control the tremors, relieve the symptoms and keep you ON.

Really the names are not important. Your doctor knows them but you must ask the questions.

What are they? How do they work? What are their benefits and side-effects?

Be informed. It will help you understand what is good for you and it is really very interesting.

Almost all of the drugs have commercial names but at the moment the one that seems best able to do the job is the combination of levodopa and carbidopa.

Simply put, the medicine is taken by mouth, goes into the digestive system and it finally gets to the brain via the blood stream. But not all of it makes it all the way.

Once there, the nerve cells convert some of it into dopamine and it starts to work to reduce the symptoms. But it also might make you a little light headed, throw up, or feel generally sick in the stomach – not good.

So it is backed up by the other drug, carbidopa. This one helps more of the levodopa get to the blood stream and stops most of the nasty little side-effects.

Up to now this is one of the best of the medical treatments in use. As the PD progresses doses might be increased or other medications used to help the brain produce more of the essential dopamine.

But your body enzymes are at work trying to stop these "invaders".

New drugs are now available to block the enzymes' attack and allow the dopamine more time and in greater amounts where it really counts - in the tiny cells of your brain. As a result you will have less "OFF" time and more "ON" times.

A lot of work is being done with a group of drugs known as dopa agonists.

Their aim is to reduce the tremor, keep rigidity to a minimum, speed you up, and help improve walking and balance.

They come most often as pills that you take either once a day or several times in smaller doses. There even is one that is delivered through a skin patch.

Sometimes the new medicines can cause unwanted problems. Your legs may swell, and your mouth and eyes might feel dry. Doses can be reduced or changed to counteract these problems.

You will need to have some good discussions with your doctor about the newer treatments and their effects but there are some really interesting new and old ideas being used.

Occasionally a new treatment is the result of a lucky find, as was the case when penicillin was discovered and was such a huge success in treating all sorts of infections.

One treatment for PD symptoms came about when a medicine used to treat influenza eased unwanted movements and tremors.

It works by helping release dopamine produced by your own brain into the system of nerve cell ends (called synapses) so it can be transmitted and shared among the other cells to reduce the symptoms.

In neurology clinics dealing with PD almost everywhere, researchers are looking for the actual site in the brain that creates the tremor and other symptoms of PD. They want to know how dopamine really works and what stops it working. They will find the answers.

More and better medical treatments are in the works and will come sooner or later. Time is your best friend in all of this so make the most of it.

The Physiotherapy Option

Contrary to popular belief, physiotherapists (commonly called physios) are not physio-terrorists.

Good physiotherapists are very well trained, highly professional, and have a very important role to play in treating the symptoms of PD. Great ones can do more for you than almost anyone else except yourself.

Search out a physio you feel comfortable with to play a key part in establishing an exercise program to help manage your PD symptoms.

Do your best to get one that is highly trained, knows about the latest PD treatments and can work with you as you are now and where you want to be.

You are a unique mixture of biology and natural machine. The physio will call this body of yours a "biomechanical chain" – which means simply that your biology, the special being that is you, and all your systems that move you around and about are linked together. A good physio will work with you on your entire body.

So, the task of the physio is to help you improve movement at all levels, control your body and counter the effect of PD at every joint, muscle and nerve system. And they can do it. Later we will see how and what that is.

Most of the symptoms of PD affect movement, balance, and control of the body.

Some words you will hear often as you visit doctors and physios are strange and technical, but you need to know them and what they mean – which is usually very easy to learn.

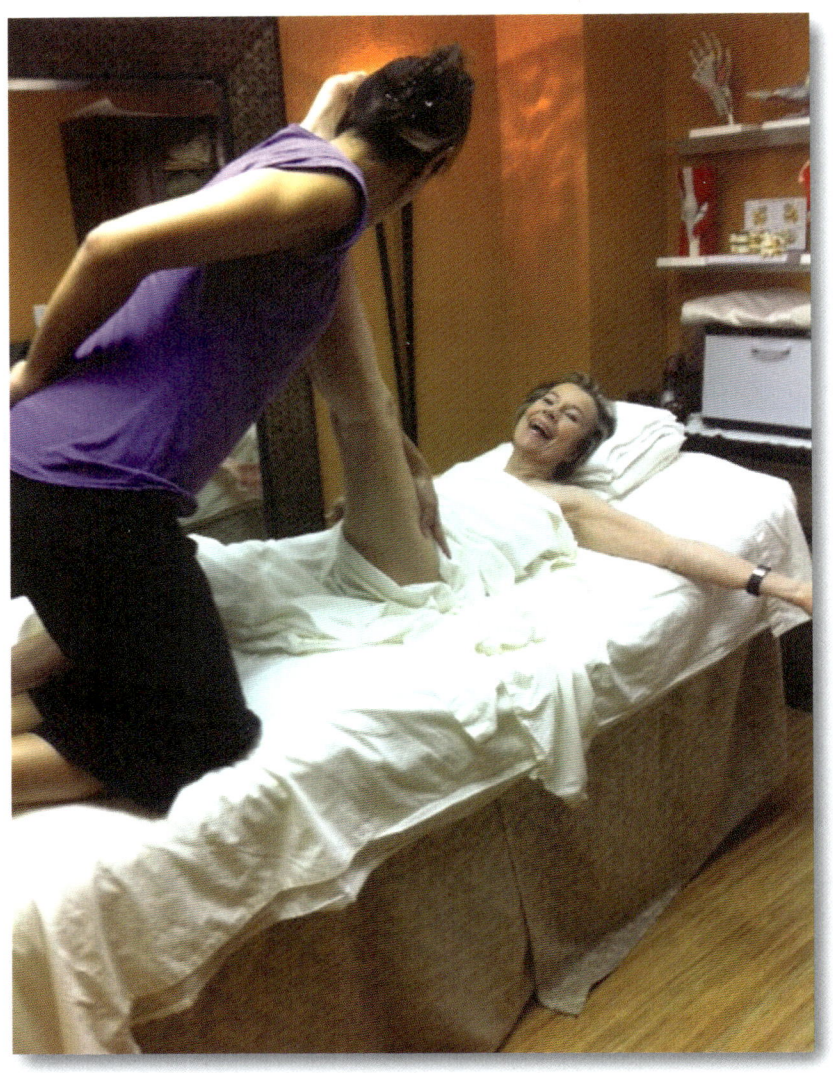

Getting to grips with your physio might look like medieval torture but it is relaxing, positive and often a load of fun. Enjoy it and benefit from it.

Your body movements have probably slowed down. It takes more time to do simple tasks. Try as you might you cannot speed things up. This is called bradykinesia.

You start rocking and rolling and writhing around but you are not at a disco, there is no music, and you were reading the paper. This is dyskinesia.

Kinesia means movement.

Sometimes movement does not happen at all, even though you want it to. That's akinesia.

Simply stated, a doctor named Brady thought up bradykinesia, and "a" means none, and the dys means more or less out of control.

It actually does not matter what they are called just so long as you know what it all means.

The Third Option – You

Sometimes, and perhaps too often, patients are treated as precisely that – patients.

But patients are people first and foremost, with hopes and problems, dreams and desires, families, friends and lovers. Each is unique in the real sense of the word. Every one is alive and, in almost every case, wanting to live.

You are one of these and you have every right and reason to continue to be a complete person, to live life in the fullest way possible, to receive the best care that can be offered, to have confidence in the present, and hope in the future.

Expect it, demand it and obtain it, especially from yourself. PD can be lived with and life can be enjoyed.

The human brain is an extremely powerful weapon that can be used for good or bad. It can create or destroy. And it is yours to control.

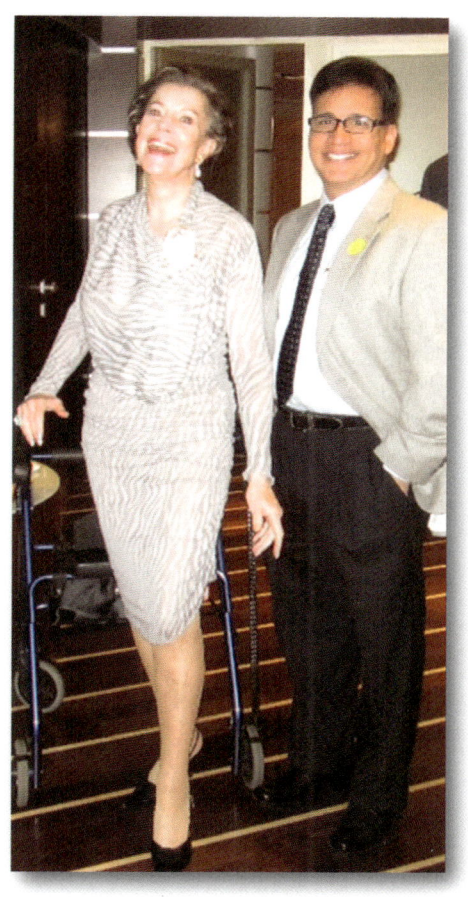

Dress as you wish to feel, control your environment and be as attractive and vibrant as you can possibly be – with or without your walker!

Same for men! People will admire you and enjoy your company.

The most important and best attack on PD is to decide your course of action and set about doing it. You will soon learn what you can do easily, what is more difficult, some tasks that are very hard, and even some that now seem impossible - without new medicine or treatment.

Next let's look at what is going to happen now that you know what the problem is.

The prognosis is much better than many other illnesses. The disease is slow and its symptoms can be treated. The future holds promising new discoveries, new treatments and increased hope.

And, best of all, you are still very much part of that future.

KNOWING PD – GETTING THE BETTER OF IT

The sad fact is that PD as yet has no cure and it is not yet known precisely what causes it or how to prevent it.

There are treatments for its symptoms as they progress and these are becoming, better, easier and more effective. Eventually a cure will be found.

The Early Years

Once the shock of the first diagnosis has been overcome and the treatment planning has commenced, it is time to look at how PD develops over time and how it can be dealt with.

The symptoms are fairly easy to observe but they do progress. The trick is to try to slow them down, knock some of them out, and take control over all that can be managed.

We have already had a brief look at the symptoms that brought you to the doctor for the diagnosis.

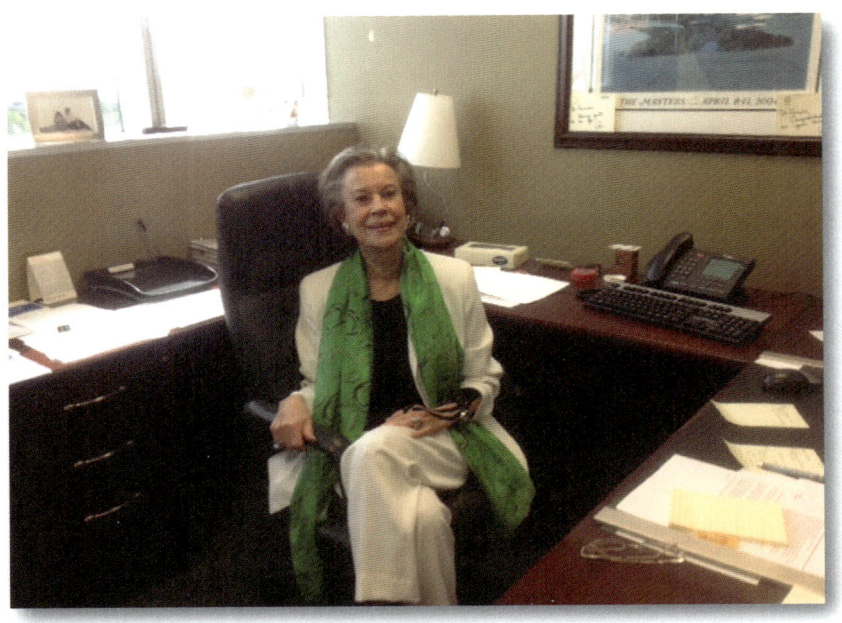

PD does not stop you from doing almost all of the daily activities that make life full and interesting. Don't retreat, stay in charge.

So let's take on that irritating and really annoying tremor first.

The tremor is likely intermittent, sometimes ever present and it is hard to stop.

It happens more often when the limb is at rest, and this is much less of a problem than when you pour the coffee down your sleeve.

Tremors can also affect the stability of the head and impair speech.

The tremor can be lessened and controlled by medication. First choice is usually a combination drug that helps the brain create dopamine and controls the side effects.

Fine finger coordination can become especially difficult, even in very familiar tasks such as buttoning a shirt, opening a screw top jar, or threading a needle.

You might be feeling happy and relaxed but your face has lost some of its mobility and you may actually look unhappy, depressed or distant although you are none of these.

Once you were a member of the High School Marching Band - all high-stepping, arm-swinging and full of martial rhythm. Now your arms don't swing, your legs drag a bit and the high steps are more like a soft shoe shuffle.

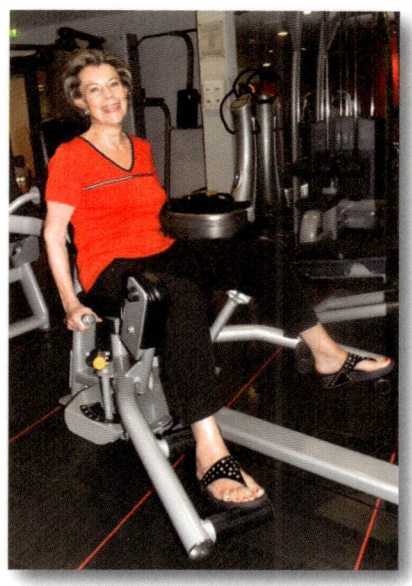

Just sit down and off you go.
But you do not need to have a gym or the machine.
You can also do this sitting in a chair at home peddling the air.
It's also great training for pedal boat racing on your favorite lake.

Your shoulder might freeze or be stiff and sore. In fact any of your limbs can be stiff or numb, and sometimes painful. Medication, physiotherapy and positive action will help.

Most of these symptoms usually start on one side of your body.

Do not despair. There is a plan, and though break dancing or life as a prima ballerina may be a thing of the past, a good gait and arms and feet under control are still possible.

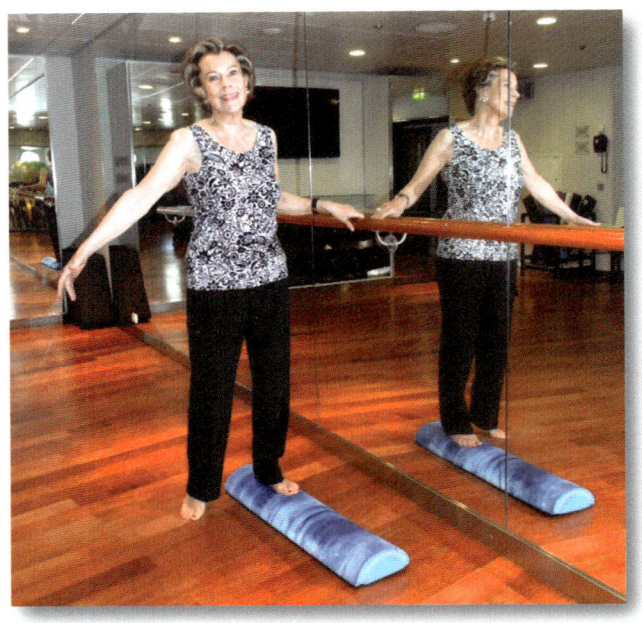

The Bolshoi beckons but you might not want to give up your day job. It's also very nice to see yourself in the mirror but you can do this one from any rail anywhere. Just make sure it doesn't come loose from the wall.

No rail? Then try your tabletop, or kitchen counter.

Today's medications will work well in almost all cases for the next 5 and possibly 10 years. Increased dosages might be needed during that time and the current medications will probably need support from other drugs in the later years.

But 10 years is a very long time in the 21st century scheme of things. Ten years ago there was no Facebook, Linkedin, iPad or X Factor. Social media did not exist and selfies were unheard of. Not all these changes are necessarily for the better!

In 10 years there will be much improved medications. New drugs will be available. New treatments will have been tested and approved. A cure or prevention might not yet be found – but a breakthrough can happen any time.

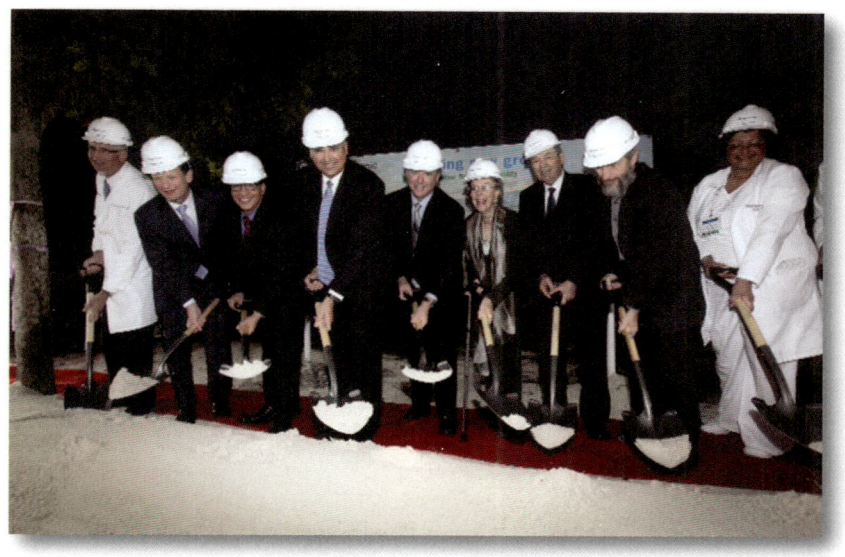

*Break new ground wherever you go.
Keep up with the latest research and treatments.
Dig into the internet and pick your doctor's brains.
Ask your phsyio to tell you what's new. Be part of the solution!*

More about the Physio Option

Drugs are usually the first treatment of choice for most of the earlier symptoms of PD but physiotherapy has a big role to play.

The physio will work with you to plan a program of exercises that you can do at home or in a gym if you have access to one. There is also hydrotherapy if you can get the use of a pool or hot tub.

Not every exercise will do what you want of it. Some will do more. But try them all and select the ones with the physio that work best for you. It is neither rocket science nor training for the Super Bowl.

Physiotherapy aims at decreasing the tremor and improving your coordination.

The physio will do a series of tests on coordination of the hands, levels of dexterity, and grip strength for example. Then a plan of exercises will be made. It will be based on specialized activities for the hands and arms.

Your arm may be held firmly or braced when the tremor is happening. Simple tasks will be given to you to improve your coordination.

Deep breathing and meditation can also steady your hands or feet. So will some strengthening and resistance training.

Most likely the physio will start your sessions off with stretching exercises.

These are nice and easy to do and very pleasant as you are lying down and stretching as many muscles as you can from head to toe. Hold onto each one for about 90 seconds or so and then do the next set.

But do stay awake!

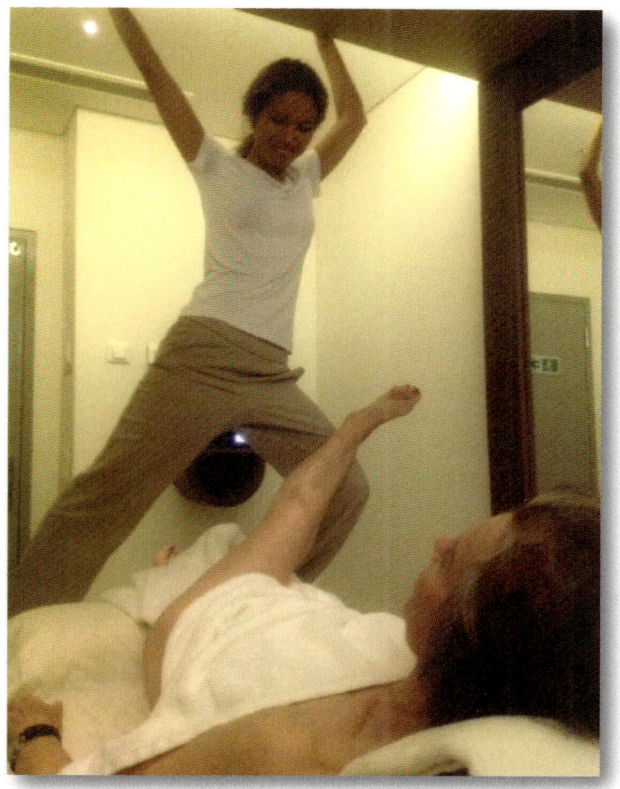

Stretching and massage is great whether you have PD or not. It feels so good when it is done and you are refreshed and renewed. Get into it and out of the bed.

You can also do this sitting up. The idea is to lengthen your muscles and keep them supple and relaxed.

Once you have mastered the technique you can even do them without the physio present. Lie on the bed, sit in a chair or lean against the wall.

The physio will probably give you a series of light massages to help the relaxation process.

Some of these techniques have the usual strange names. One is called Myofascial Release.

The muscles in your body are connected, protected and supported by a tissue. The soft part of this tissue is the fascia.

Your physio will use a massage technique to work on the fascia to relax contracted muscles, improve blood and lymphatic circulation, and stimulate the stretching reflex.

It feels good and does work.

Do not go into a terror spasm if the physio mentions that he or she is doing a "cranial sacral" on you. Your skull is not being shrunken and no human sacrifice witch doctors are present.

Your physio will touch or press the hands against your skull, face, spine, and even your pelvis, quite softly, so that you feel very relaxed, and sometimes even a bit lightheaded.

There are many more treatments available to a well-trained physio. Learn about them and find the ones that work best for you.

Ask questions and get answers.

None of it is painful or difficult to do and it can help a lot.

Pauline really likes this option. She never misses her gym sessions and she has a complete range of exercises made especially for her. Your physio will do the same for you.

"It is not hard, but it is consistent", Pauline says, "You must do it as planned, regularly and with a real sense of purpose. It is made for you and it will work for you, just as it does for me.

Sometimes I get very tired but I always feel better for having done the exercises."

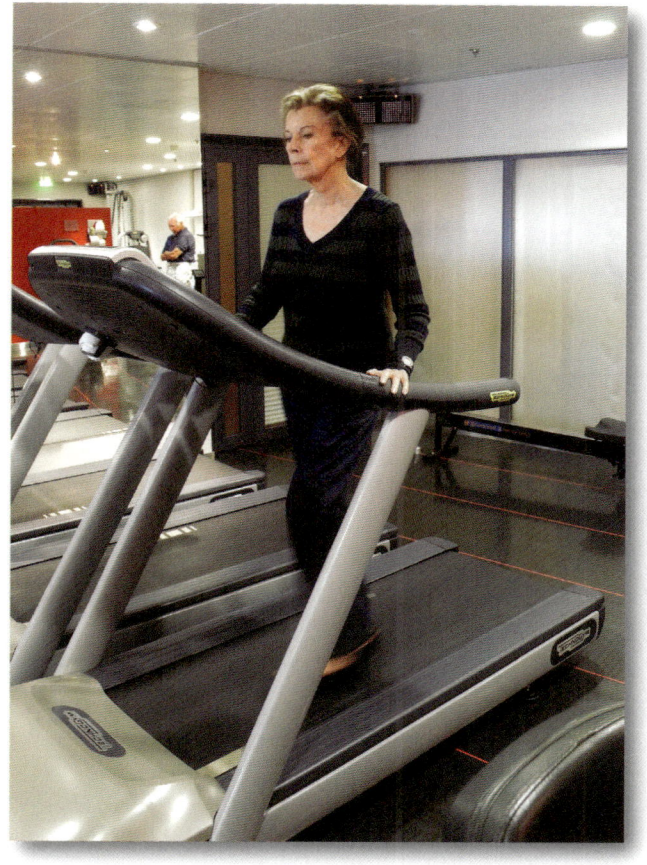

*This one is not bad either.
You walk on the machine and it walks with you.
It is not so easy to keep smiling on it. All gyms have treadmills.
Stationary bikes are not expensive either and can give
you lots of good exercise right at home.*

Pauline's experience is a very good guide to what can be tried and how it works.

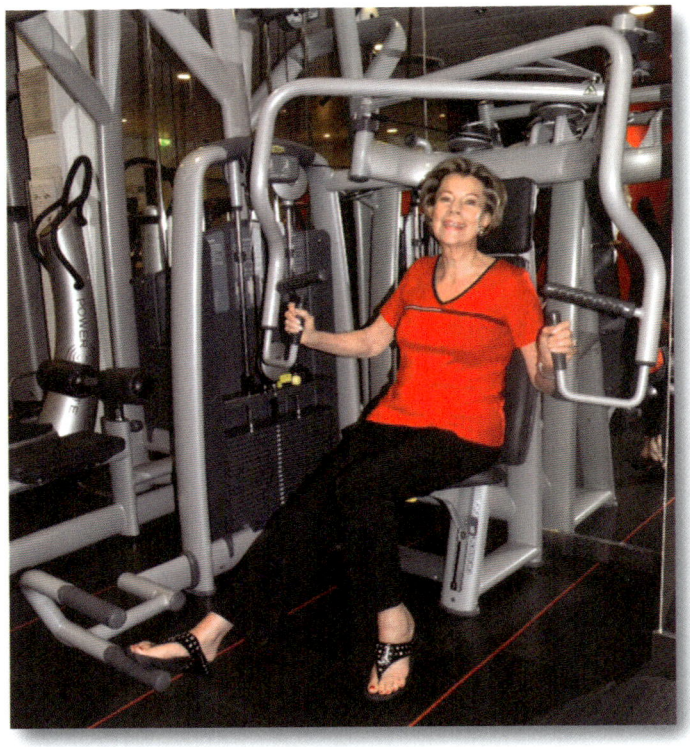

You will really like using this machine - it does all sorts of things for your arms and upper body and all you do is sit in it and push it around.

"The physiotherapy program focuses on stretching, massage, and manual manipulation. It has worked so well that I continue to eat without any help and conduct my everyday normal tasks unworried about the tremors, although they still occur.

"The massage is great, even if you haven't got PD, but you can live without it and just do the exercises.

"But you must really do them – they are one of your best ways to control that shaky feeling and keep it at arms length!"

PD is much more than a tremor in the arm or other parts of your body. If your gait is affected, or if you feel you might tumble over backwards, or you are thinking of buying an elevator or stair lift, then help is needed.

The old standby, ever researched, renewed, and always more beneficial as time goes by, is medication. Increased doses, new medicines and drug options continue to be developed, tested and made available.

But with or without medication, physiotherapy can be really helpful.

Once again there will be tests to create a personalized plan. This time it is more intensive and wide ranging.

You are likely to be tested for your range of motion, the length of your muscles, your reflexes and other parts of your nervous system.

Balance analysis is essential, especially to assess your risk of falling.

Some of your muscle groups might be observed via EMG while they are working, or you might become a TV star on a treadmill as the video camera captures the way you walk at different levels and speeds.

Once the evaluation has been done a new plan will be created. It is more extensive than the first series on the hands and arms and concentrates more on the legs and lower body.

It might not get you to the Olympics but it will knock PD back a step or two.

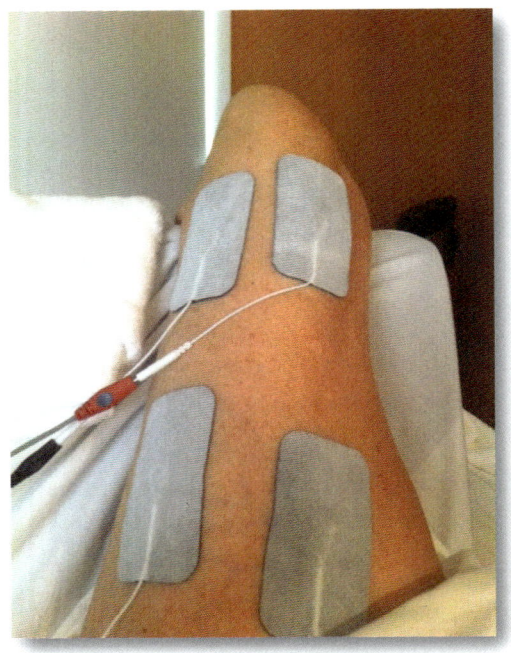

Showing a leg like this might not be the ultimate turn-on, but the action can still be electric.

Balance training will play a big part.

This will include exercises to get your weight shifting back and forward and also diagonally. You might use parallel bars, the treadmill or mechanical support systems to help you steady your walking patterns – or gait.

If you are a dancer or like rhythms you will probably enjoy the rhythm sessions that invite you to march to a different beat.

And you will get back that long loping stride, or part of it anyway.

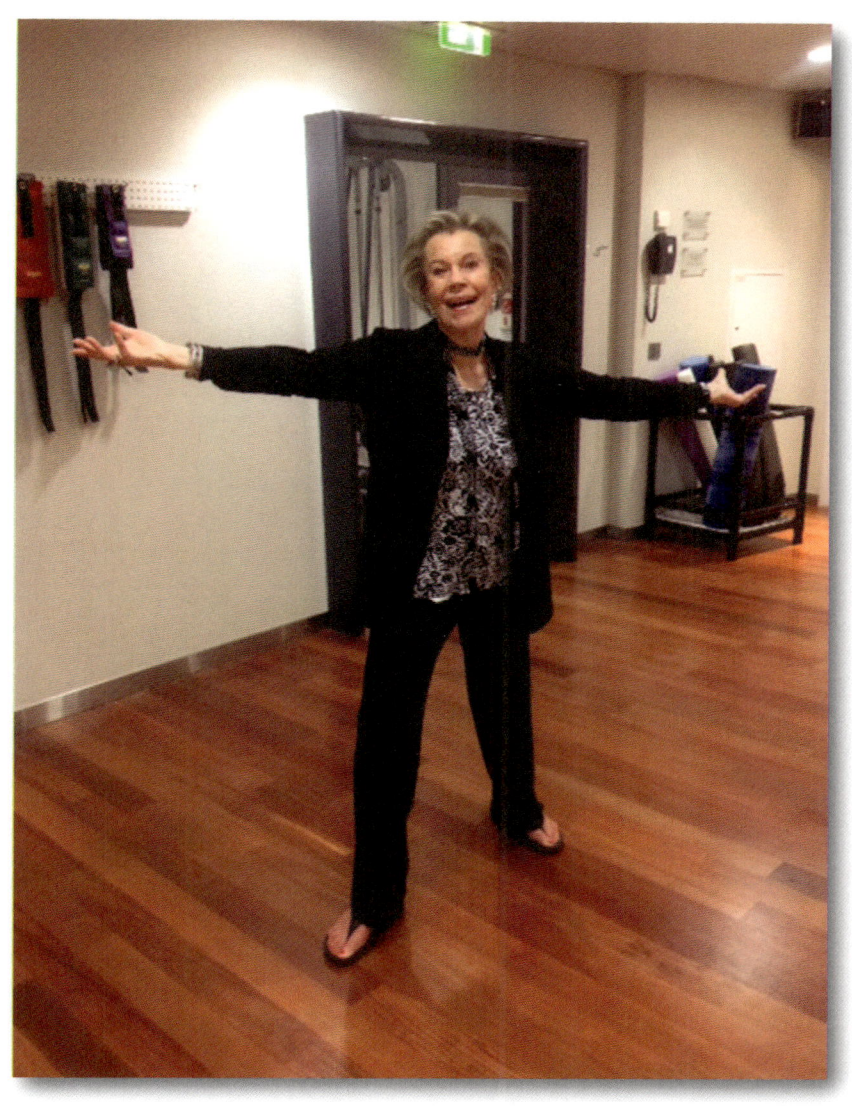

*Stride out like a dancer and stretch your legs out as far as you can. Keep them flexible and use your arms as well.
It is your body and you can make it work for you.*

WHAT HAPPENS AFTER 5-10 YEARS WITH PD?

OK – So what next?

If you were diagnosed with PD a few years ago you will not be reading this. You will already be involved with the medications and treatments that are in place now and that were developed in the time since you were diagnosed and today.

But if you got the diagnosis in the last twelve months or two years and your PD is in its early stages you have much good news to look forward to.

Tried and tested medications already exist to help control the symptoms as the disease progresses.

All the therapies continue to improve as more and more is learned about PD and its effects on a large number of people.

And consider this:

If the progress made in the last ten years is even simply matched in the next decade you may never reach the more advanced stages.

Your symptoms will be more effectively treated and controlled. The medicines will have reduced side effects, the dopamine-producing agents will be more reliable and better controlled - delivering more and needing less.

It may be too much to hope for a cure in ten years but it is possible and it can happen.

Think back to breast or prostate cancer 10 years ago, or almost any cancer from that era. Most have much greater survivability than could even have been dreamed of then.

Consider HIV and Aids even from 15 years ago and see how new treatments have saved so many lives since then. The prevention of infection by HIV might not be far off.

And you have so much more time!

So let's look into both the present and the future and see what can be done to get you to and through that ten-year time span.

Assuming that the PD progresses and that you have taken the medication and done the exercises and that everything in ten years is the same as it is today, here is what might be happening to you 5 to 10 years from now.

In some few cases it comes earlier than expected and if it does then this is what you will experience and how you can handle it.

Motor Fluctuations

You could be having motor fluctuations, which has nothing to do with your automobile.

Motor fluctuations are problems with your own movements. These are often unpredictable, occurring suddenly and disappearing just as quickly.

You can have "ON" periods when you are completely mobile to "OFF" periods where movement of any type will be difficult and occasionally impossible. It can feel like a curtain coming down and then rising again.

Treatment will mean adjusting the dose of your medication and adding other drugs that your doctor will prescribe to create a treatment cocktail – but without the olive.

Freezing

Putting yourself on ice is not the answer to dealing with PD. But your body may freeze on you without warning and certainly without your approval.

Freezing happens when you simply cannot start a task as simple as getting out of a chair. Your feet seem to be stuck to the floor with superglue. It may even affect your speech so that starting a sentence just does not happen.

It is not yet known how and why this occurs.

Some researchers think there may be another problem with the nerves transmitting chemicals other than dopamine. Perhaps it is morphine-like substances that occur naturally in the body. But no one really knows. So there is no medication available yet that is of any real help.

But do not despair. The clever physios in collaboration with patients like Pauline have learned ways to trick PD and fool the body into defrosting.

Trade the laptop for an iPod and start listening to music with a strong rhythmic beat.

Get the frozen movement in your gait to listen to it too.

If you can borrow or buy a metronome set it going when you are moving around the house. Listen to its regular tick and pattern it into your walk. It's the beat, beat, beat of the drum that keeps that old black magic in your steps.

Tap on your leg or hip in time with the beat and the chances are your legs and hips and whatever other parts are frozen will warm up and begin to work.

If you are older than 60 put your "ol' blue eyes" record on and walk to his *New York, New York*.

If you do not know who "ol' blue eyes" was then use Michael Jackson or Lady Gaga or whoever turns your dancing feet on.

If you have no access to music-players start tapping with your cane or a wooden spoon, or start singing or counting, or do anything you can to create a strong rhythm - and then start moving.

It can also look pretty hip to your kids when you groove into the beat.

Getting up from a chair can be a challenge. Try lifting your knees up in turn around 10 times each, and then rock back and forth 5 or 6 times in the chair. This will help you get moving and get up.

Most often the freeze will occur when you are moving from one position to another, such as from sitting to standing or lying down, or even from standing to walking. So work to the rhythm, do the exercises and keep on doing them.

If you have access to a pool or deep hot tub remember that water exercises are really helpful, and so easy to do.

Walk forward, backwards and sideways. Lift your knees as high as you can and, if you are feeling really energized, jump up and down in the water bending your knees as you go.

A walker with balanced wheels and brakes will help to unfreeze the legs and produce a smooth gait.

Pauline has a cool silver cane and an ever-ready walker to beat these symptoms and rarely needs a wheelchair to get herself to where she wants to be.

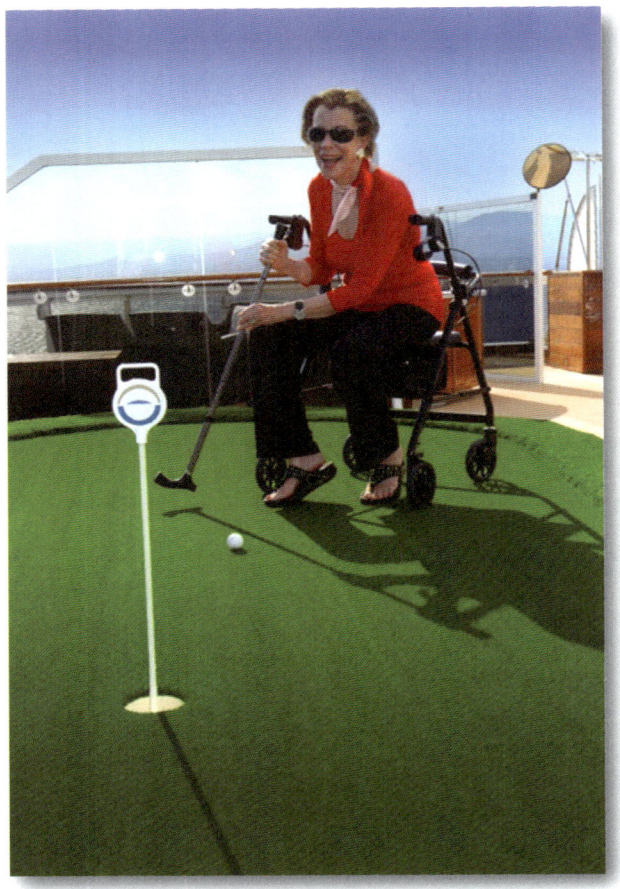

*My first game of golf was not quite like the Masters,
but it was really quite a laugh.
The walker and the putter seemed made for each other.
Think of it as a self-propelled buggy.*

Much more can be done to move the body into motion.

If the problem has not been solved by the researchers in the years to come and by the time you get there, then you can also try some of these tricks to keep that tortoise to a very slow crawl.

Push down as hard as you can on the frozen foot and then lift it straight up.

Rock back and forth heel to toe.

Bend and then straighten the knees.

Bring your arms out and up in short quick movements.

Try kicking your cane, or the wastebasket, or anything else in range. It might not work but it will make you feel good. Just don't kick the cats - they do not like it and may not want to visit you for a while!

A friend or family member is often a very helpful ally to counter-attack freezing.

They should touch you lightly to guide you – never pulling or pushing – and they can lead you gently by having you imitate their movements. Do not kick them either.

All distractions should be minimized. It is much better to continue moving without stopping.

Invent your own tricks to deceive the body, confuse PD and freeze it in its own tracks.

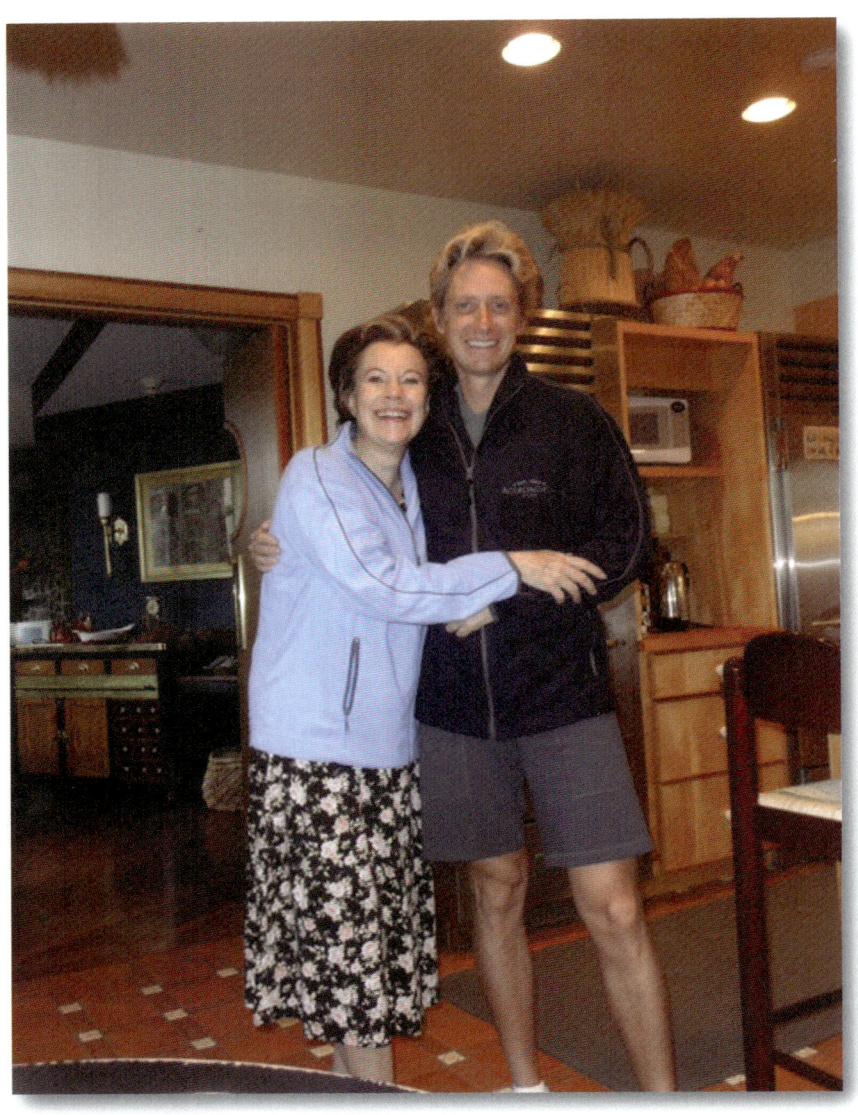

*This is a little more like it! Being helped by good friends is a pleasure if you accept it and let them enjoy doing it.
A good old-fashioned cuddle does no harm either.*

Swallowing

Way in the future, maybe 10 to 20 years on, you might begin to have problems swallowing. Which is not great if you like food and want to continue to eat.

But there are good ways to overcome this and some of them may be better for you anyway.

First off - eat smaller but more frequent meals. Order half portions in restaurants. Cut the food into small bite size bits and chew them well. Have a sip of a favorite drink after each swallow – use a straw if you find it helps.

Soft foods go down easier than hard varieties – chicken, ground meats, soups, stews – there is a huge range to chose from.

Keep the food warm – not too hot or cold.

Sit up when eating, chin to chest when swallowing.

Swallow several times before the next forkful. Make sure the first lot is well and truly down where it should be.

Just in case everything seizes up and you start turning a little bluish, make sure all your family members and the friends you like to dine with can do the Heimlich manoeuvre.

You may lose your teeth and whatever you swallowed, but at least you will be there for dessert.

Think about your diet and plan ahead whenever you can. Let your friends know what you can eat easily and which foods are hard to swallow.

Talk to a dietician about the best way to get all the nutrition you need from food you can enjoy without fear of getting it down.

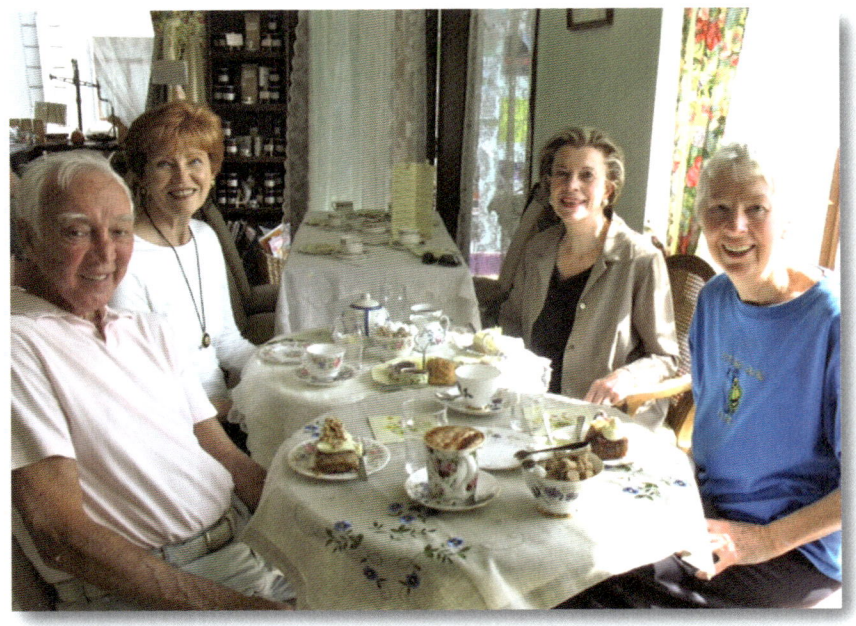

*Enjoy the food, the company and the ambience.
Do not worry if you eat slowly or sometimes have to stop.
Everyone will understand. Good friends together in a lovely teashop is priceless.*

Speaking Softly

You are beginning to think your friends and family are losing their hearing.

Before you suggest a good set of hearing aids you might have to consider a problem common to PD called hypophonia – loss of volume when speaking.

This can be really irritating in a noisy restaurant when the waiter cannot hear your order or your friends give up trying to guess what you are wanting to say. It is bad anywhere there is any sort of noise.

You need to make the most of what volume you can muster.

Before you start speaking get your thoughts in order so that you can make your point clearly and briefly.

Make sure your dentures are firmly in place and swallow any unwanted saliva.

Take a deep breath. Then start firmly and clearly – you do not have to sound like someone from *Downton Abbey*, but clear diction will greatly help you and your friends to enjoy the conversation.

Exaggerate if you need to. Make your facial muscles work and be expressive with your face, hands and body language. It can be great fun.

Keep sentences short.

If it is too noisy, wait for a quieter place and time. Most people talk too much anyway and this is a good time for you to be brief, concise and be taken very seriously.

You can also work on your tongue action and your lip and jaw muscles with a speech therapist.

Talk into a recorder and play it back. Work always to improve the diction and be as clear and precise as possible.

You might not regain the volume you once had but your friends and family may actually listen harder and be more attentive than ever before.

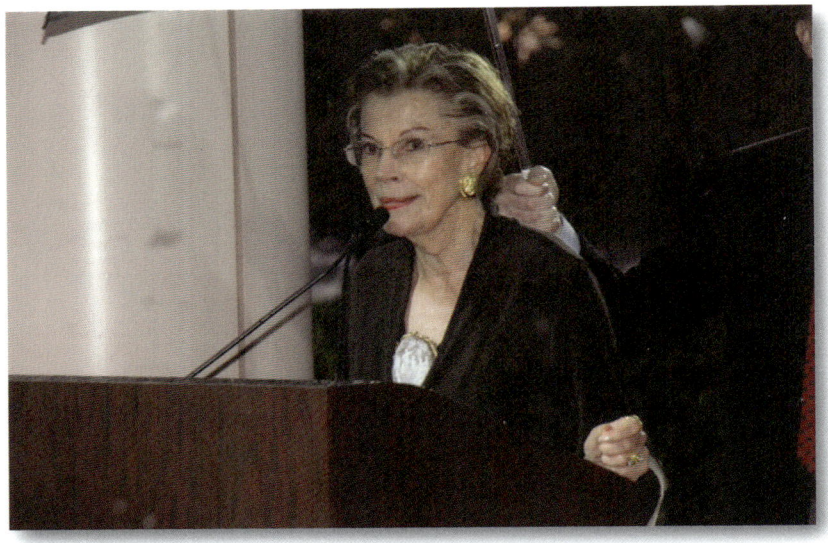

Speak softly and command attention. If you like acting, speaking and being a bit of a star attraction go for it all. Learn to use a mike and speak as clearly as you can.

NERVOUS SYSTEM NUISANCES

Some of these are not great. They include such little and large evils as constipation, frequent bathroom visits, light headedness, hallucinations and even impotence.

Taking Viagra probably won't be a good idea for the last of these.

Constipation in PD is different from the hard going that results from bad foods or poor diets. It is most likely caused by the autonomic nervous system, that part of your nervous system that automatically functions without you having to think about it. Now you do!

The autonomic nervous system regulates the movements of your digestive system – the gastrointestinal tract. PD is thought to slow this movement down and constipation is the result.

You can take medications that soften the stool, or that purge the bowels, or even fill the tract with lots of bulk.

But you may be better off if you think more about establishing consistent eating patterns and trying to keep your toilet visits regular as well.

Increase the amount of natural fibre you eat – whole grain breads and rice are very good. Raw fruits and leafy vegetables will help you to go, so will bran-based cereals, lentils, split peas and barley. Prunes are a natural laxative but be careful – they can work very quickly and explosively.

Drink plenty of water, as many as 8 glasses a day if you can. Exercise often and at least once every day. Try Senna tea. A nightly glass of hot water or cool prune juice can loosen things up.

Bladders that won't hold water are very depressing.

There are many causes of this problem including infections, childbirth difficulties, or an enlarged prostate gland. None of these is very pleasant but nor are they the result of PD.

PD causes bladder problems without any help from the others.

Bathroom visits are too frequent, it is hard to empty the bladder completely and there is an embarrassing tendency to dribble.

So take some action here.

Limit the amount you drink at night. Stay clear of caffeine-loaded drinks, especially coffee, cola, tea and Red Bull. Even grapefruit juice will set you off.

Play it safe – keep a bedpan or commode near the bed for those quickfire emergencies.

If you don't like the smell of the urine (who does?) drink some cranberry juice daily. Just like asparagus it will "perfume" the urine, but much more pleasantly. Tastes good, too.

There are medications you can take but it is best to talk to a urologist and get up to the minute advice on what is best for you – and ask about side effects.

But! You might not be able to smell the urine, or taste the cranberry juice, or that fine wine quite so easily as before.

Your partner says the room smells like a forest full of lilies. Maybe you put your perfume on a little lavishly or overdid the aftershave.

If the kitty litter needs changing or the dog needs a wash or the smoke alarm goes bananas and you've not smelled any of it, then PD is at work.

It is insidious and slow, but it happens, although not always.

So enjoy your days of wine and roses to the full. The memories are great, even if your taste buds and nose are not what they once were.

Lightheadedness becomes a common symptom of PD as the disease progresses.

It is usually caused by not enough blood flow to the brain. It comes after a long period of PD that may by then be having an effect on blood pressure. It can also be a side effect of your medication.

You could feel as if you are going to faint and topple over. Occasionally you might. But you will wake up. Just don't do it while bungee jumping or rock climbing.

Review and check on what you are taking. Talk this over with your doctor because a reduction in the medication may strengthen the other symptoms of PD.

If it is causing you problems at night try lifting up the head end of the bed with some blocks under the legs (the bed's, not yours).

You can also increase the amount of salt you use, drink more fluids, move your arms, legs and upper body before standing, and get up slowly.

Not so much fun is avoiding alcohol and hot showers or baths, wearing support hose, and not dancing with the stars.

Impotence can be a problem for some with PD. It is likely to be associated with low blood pressure or the medication, or it can be caused by a lot of non-PD factors, so don't necessarily blame the PD for it. Best to take this one to the specialists and see what they recommend.

Neuropsychiatric Problems

This sounds awful.

Medicine loves big long terms for many conditions. This one means that something is happening in the brain cells which is affecting your ability to behave "normally" – the way you used to think and act and what people see as "normal".

PD might cause you to have mood swings, hallucinations, delusions, very vivid dreams, or be confused at times and lose your memory on and off. It may actually change your behavior towards yourself, your loved ones and your friends.

None of this is desirable in the least so first let's know what it means and then see what can be done about it.

Remember that this is almost always down the line in the advance of PD and we are determined to manage that advance by every means possible.

Mood swings are unpredictable but you can recognize them. In the old drug culture words they would have been called uppers and downers.

Uppers are sometimes called manias or manic, a term we do not much like because it has nasty side tones like manic-depressive.

You are not manic with PD, but you might be overly active, aggressive and difficult to keep still or quiet.

This will cause great concern to everyone around you. It will come and go just like your "ON" and "OFF" periods.

When this mood goes it might be replaced by a really down feeling, a depression in which all things seem to have no good in them – especially yourself.

This too will pass.

You are not "bipolar". You are feeling the effects of PD and it is no fault of yours.

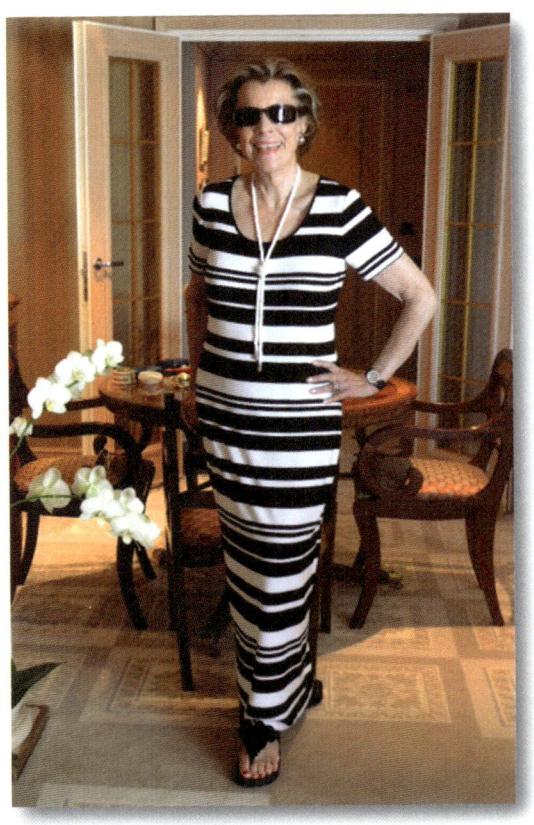

*Get dressed and go to the beach or to a restaurant or just feel good about being at home.
When you feel really down remember that very old song "Puttin' on the Ritz".*

If you can recognize the mood swings early and when they begin, whichever way they swing, you can put your own brain to work to counter them.

Counseling from a professional can help and so can medication, but sometimes the best way is to understand that this is not your doing and you are not "psychotic".

Do not blame yourself. It is the workings of the PD in its more advanced stage, so let's try to get there very slowly indeed, or not at all. Mood swings are not inevitable.

Hallucinations are by definition rather weird and unreal. A great many people without hallucinations would like to have them and pay lots of cash for various drugs, mostly illegal, just to experience the sensation.

You get them for free.

But unless they are great, exciting, joyful, full of enhanced colors and sounds, and super brilliant, you really don't want them. Getting high this way is not great fun!

There is a new generation of medicines now available that help to control the hallucinations you do not like having.

They have another of those strange names. This lot is called "atypical neuroleptics". They also help to calm things down if you get a bit over agitated when the scam callers ring in the middle of the night, or sometimes for no reason at all.

Pauline does not worry much about the names of the drugs or their technical terms. She knows them because she always asks – and so should you – what they do and how they work and what other effects they might have.

People who are not present may appear and be friendly or threatening.

Scenes that do not exist in reality become three-dimensional and you are present in them.

Almost any form of hallucination is possible – and all seem very real indeed.

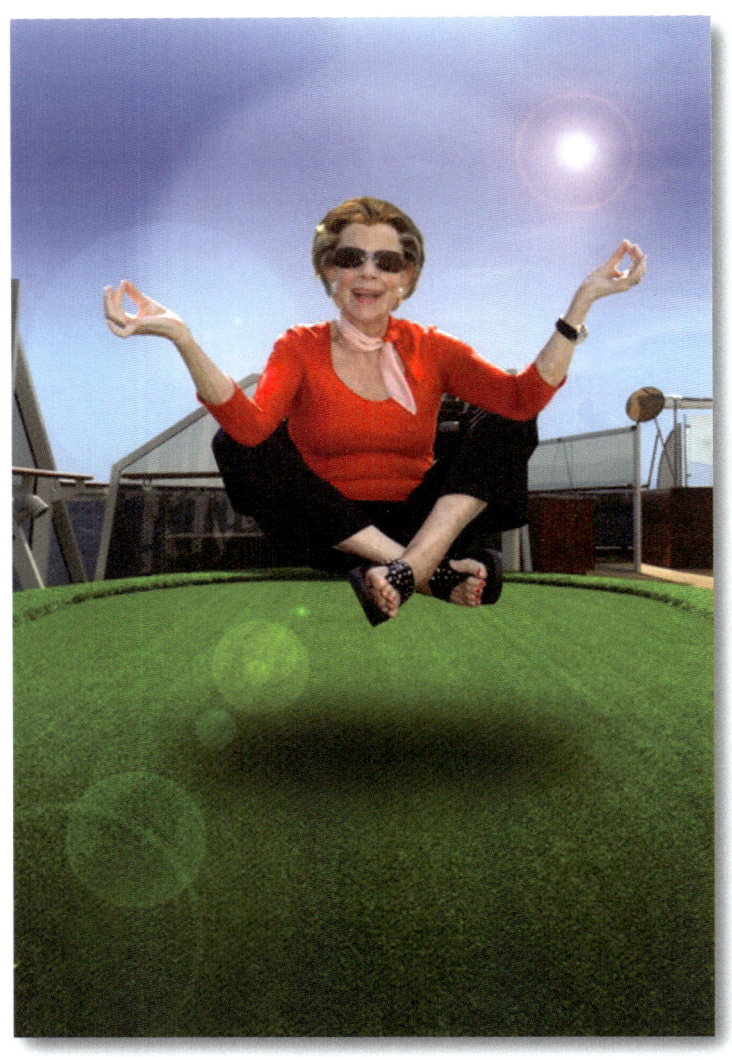

*You do not have to get high on or off grass.
Just enjoy yourself and be yourself.
Hallucinations are not for you.
If they come along unwanted there are good treatments for them.*

Delusions are also possible.

It can be a boost to your ego to believe you are God, or the President, or a great pianist or artist.

It is less fun to think that the CIA, the FBI or Scotland Yard have you on their Top Wanted Lists.

Even worse – you might believe your partner is cheating on you, your bank manager has stolen your pension, and your heirs are planning to eliminate you.

Most of these and any others are highly unlikely. But just in case, check on what you have been doing lately, take your partner to a romantic dinner, review your pension statements, and don't drink that warm milk the kids made for you to help you sleep - just kidding.

Vivid dreams used to be fun.

Sometimes they were so good that waking up was a disappointment. Not so now.

These dreams can be caused by the medication, either the ones controlling the symptoms or others working on the side effects.

Hallucinations, delusions and dreams are not funny. They can cause a lot of distress and be very confusing. But if you can treat them like any other imposters and recognize them for what they are, then you have a better chance of taking control of them.

Most often they are related to the continuing progress of PD and also, sadly, to the medications used to slow the symptoms. Really good consultations with your doctor are essential to modify doses, look at alternatives, and work against their onset.

Confusion comes with PD in its later stages. It, too, can be worsened by the very medications that are helping you and much work is being done to find other newer drugs that will not have these effects.

It can also be the result of your thyroid not producing well, or a lack of vitamin B12. Even dehydration can create confusion. Other possibilities are infections of the bladder and the urinary system, pneumonia and other illnesses.

It might also be the onset of dementia – which is not what anyone wants.

Dementia comes most often as a result of Alzheimer's disease, which is not PD. If you are diagnosed with dementia in the early stages of PD it is almost certainly not caused by the PD itself but by something else.

Dementia in PD usually appears in older people after many years of PD symptoms.

Even then your chances of avoiding it are pretty good as less than three in ten wind up with some moderate form and more often it is less than one in ten who have it to a greater degree.

Dementia produces permanent memory problems, thinking is impaired and the ability to work and be an active part of society might be lost.

Very similar but worse than confusion, PD based dementia is thought to be caused by low thyroid performance, shortage of Vitamin B12 and other illnesses. These can be treated and the dementia slowed.

Many PD patients will find that their thinking processes are changing but it rarely affects day-to-day activities.

If you sometimes have problems with depth perception, or feel disoriented, or are a little slower sizing things up, it might be wise to stop driving and to limit your jet skiing, rock climbing or skate boarding.

As always there are medications that will help. Make sure you ask about them and understand what they do.

New ones will always be coming on stream and they will be ever better at doing their job as the years go by.

The bad news is that none of them, so far, cures PD or makes the tortoise crawl much more slowly. But they will stop or reduce the symptoms, and that is the good news.

Remember, your problem is not Alzheimer's. It is PD and it is ever so slow moving. Keep on top of it and you can help delay the onset of all of these neuropsychiatric problems.

Make that tortoise work for every inch of ground.

REVISITING THE THIRD OPTION – YOU

Well there you are.

You have PD but you have it under control with medication and exercise and knowledge. You know it is no sprinter and you are keeping it to a minimal crawl.

You and your doctor and physio are making PD earn every advance it makes and stopping some of them cold.

Now what can you do to make the best of every moment of every day? How can you set up your life to be independent of the problems caused by PD, or at least minimize the effects of them?

Action is much better than passivity!

Attitude

Gloom and doom is an option. Not a good one and it won't help you much.

Denial is another, equally useless, although it may give you a little short-term relief.

Excessive optimism is better than the first two options but it won't last and may result in deeper and gloomier feelings.

You control your thoughts.

But you now have a realistic understanding of PD, recognizing that it is very slow in its harmful effects.

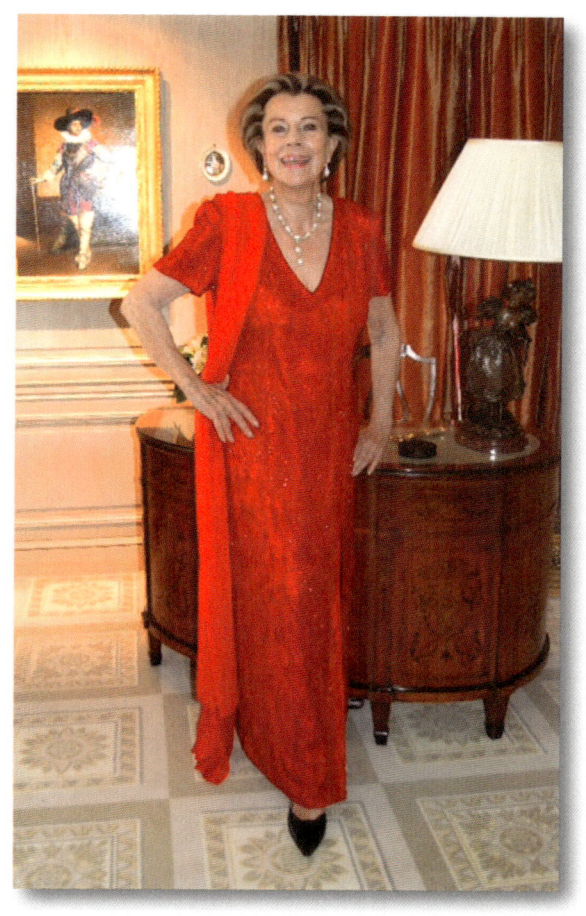

*Dress up and be as glamorous as you can be. It makes you feel
good and it keeps you younger than your years.
But that is not always for everyone...
Woman or man, it is all the same.
Don't let PD wear you down, challenge it all the way
and keep it at bay until that cure is found.*

There are good treatments and therapies in place now, and extremely dedicated and talented people are working daily with ever-increasing knowledge and resources to control, contain and eventually to defeat PD.

The best option of all is to use this knowledge to make the most of every day. Enjoy the things that you can do well and share your positive thinking with your family and friends.

It can be done and you can do it.

See what Pauline has done to make life good, even great, while handling PD and keeping its progress to a minimum.

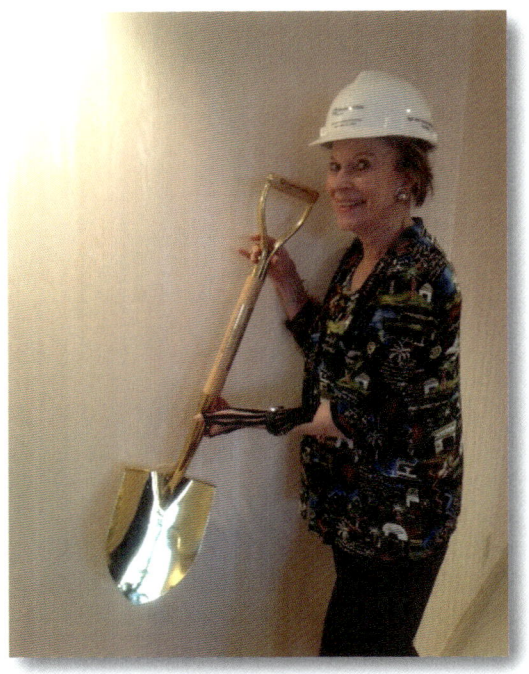

Hard hats and spades are great for show, but attitude is for real, even if you have to brace yourself occasionally!
PD is no pushover and at times the going will be hard, but a positive attitude will help you immensely over the rougher spots in the road.

ORGANIZING YOUR ENVIRONMENT

Look around your home and at how you live. Think about what you can do in your environment to make being alive safer, easier and better.

Balance and walking might already be a problem, so eliminate those slippery rugs and mats or, if you love them greatly, get non skid backs put on them.

Skating out of control across the living room floor is a no-fun and undesirable activity.

Put safety rails along corridors and up stairways. Use them.

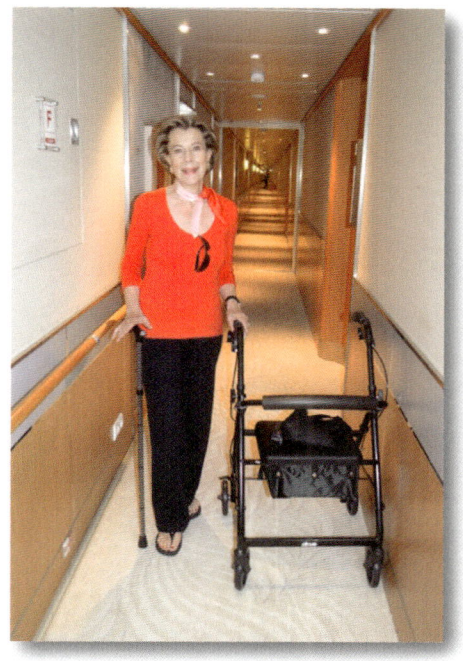

Make a friend of your walker (not the two-legged escort variety). Use the safety rails and don't forget the stick that steadies you. You might not need either of these if you are recently diagnosed, but they are great supporters and will not let you down.

If standing up in the shower is unsteady, get a nice comfortable stool or chair and relax. You can use a lower one in the bath too and it will help you get in and out of the tub.

If the toilet seat is difficult to get down to or up from, get a higher one installed, or add circular cushions to it (with the mandatory hole of course).

Make yourself secure and comfortable but do not doze off. Falling off the seat will definitely not be a good thing.

Electric toothbrushes and razors work very well and need much less fine finger control.

Rubber grips on hand held toothbrushes are good for gripping, but not many safety razors are designed for PD users.

Slippery soap is a nuisance for everyone, a lurking hazard for anyone with PD. Try soap on a rope or get liquid soap dispensers installed.

If you are finding difficulty in getting to personal places you want to gently scrub or wash, a long handled soft brush, or a big sponge or toweling mitts will all help, and will feel good too.

Do it yourself, or have someone you like do it for you. You don't have to stop having fun.

Cleaning the house will probably get harder. Use tools that help such as longer handled dusters and easy to use vacuums.

In the kitchen try to install Lazy Susans so you can easily reach equipment, jars or whatever it is you want.

Have aprons made with extra large pockets, your hands will thank you for this.

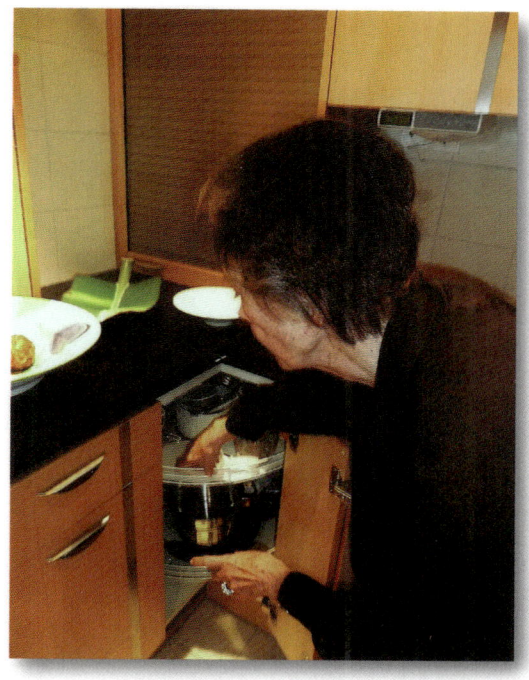

*Make it easy on yourself.
Your Lazy Susan can be a very hard worker to help ease the strains of everyday living.
Keep your jars and kitchen wear within easy reach.*

If you can't load or unload the dishwasher (this should not happen for a very long time) or if you do not have one, attach a spray hose to the sink tap to help clean plates and cutlery easier and better.

It is time for bed, and sometimes it is not as great a place to be as the soap operas would like us believe.

This is especially so when you have PD. But much can be done to get a better night's sleep and really enjoy it.

If your bed sheets seem to be made of Velcro or horsehair and won't let you turn easily, buy a pair of satin ones. They have a lovely sheen and you can slide easily on them.

Also you will look and feel good on, or in, the satin sheets, which does no harm to the self-image.

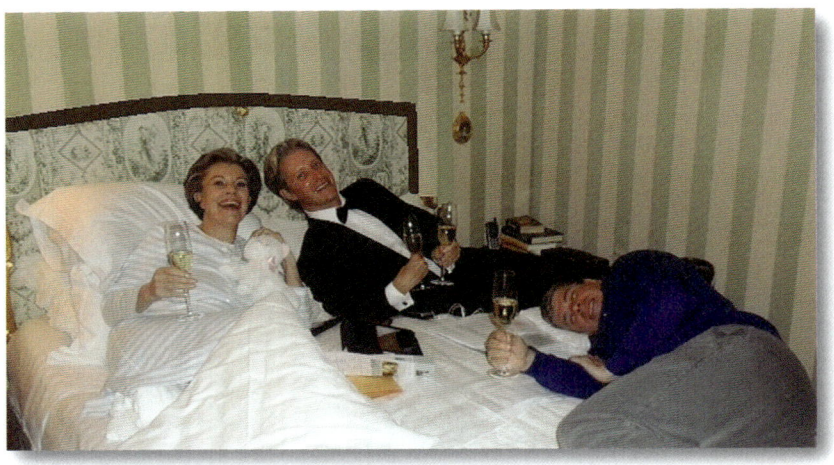

Well, it was New Year's Eve, after midnight, and everyone was very friendly and relaxed! Come out of your shell. Enjoy the life you have, especially when you are "ON" - as everyone is in this one.

If you have trouble getting out of bed you could think about installing a rope above it and then you can use your arm strength, or raise the head of the bed so you can get gravity to help.

Clear away obstructions that might cause you to trip, place chairs and dressers in easy reach in case you need to steady yourself. Do not have anything on rollers that can take you on an unwanted ride. Know the layout of everything.

There are many ways you can make your home safer and easier to live in with PD.

Take it upon yourself to design your space so you are totally comfortable living in it.

You know yourself best of all, so trust yourself first.

BEING ACTIVE

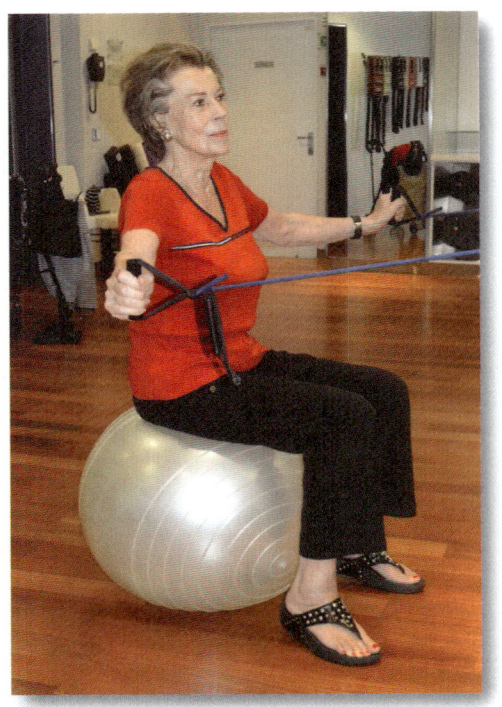

*Balance, movement and stretching.
Easy to do and oh so valuable to keep you supple,
strong and mobile. Have a ball!*

Mobility, power and endurance - three key elements of life affected by PD.

Mobility is paramount, power is necessary, and endurance helps you stay in the game. What can you do to enhance, protect and prolong these essential three?

Mobility is helped by simply stretching and moving every muscle group you have.

Moving rhythmically and swinging your arms naturally whenever and wherever you can are great for mobility, even if people think you might be a little strange – ignore them.

Move as well as you can every time you have the chance. If you have access to a pool you can develop a mobility exercise program with the help of your physio or even a fitness trainer.

You do not need to swim if you can't. Work out in the shallow end.

The water helps to take the shock away from the joints and allows you to move much more freely. All good physios know how to make a program that will suit your needs.

Slow, controlled exercises like Tai Chi are very popular and there are others you can try. Find which ones you enjoy doing and do them whenever you can.

Power needs constant help

Weight training (with dumbbells not diets) is good for this. But keep the weights light and do lots of repetitions.

You won't need expensive equipment or a gym if there isn't one nearby. Two cans of soup - one in each hand - will work well enough to get started.

It is much better if you can use a gym or fitness centre where you can talk with the physio or a fitness trainer and set up a regular schedule of exercises for weight training and power retention.

Personalized programs are usually very much more effective than haphazard attempts or home grown ones. More and better physios are being trained in helping the PD person and, always, the knowledge base increases.

Endurance must be maintained. You need it to keep going and outpacing PD. It is the easiest to work on.

It is easy because it's as simple as walking as much as you can and as briskly as possible. It can be enhanced by swimming and water exercises. If you feel comfortable riding a bike then do it.

If you think you might tumble off a two-wheeler then use a stationary bike at home or in the gym. Risk taking is not a great option.

Rowing machines, treadmills, zumba classes – all can help improve endurance and most are fun.

If you like to dance and can disco, quickstep, salsa, samba or rumba, go for it. It is one of your best activities to keep fit and enjoy life.

Or try some kick boxing – it's great for releasing aggression!

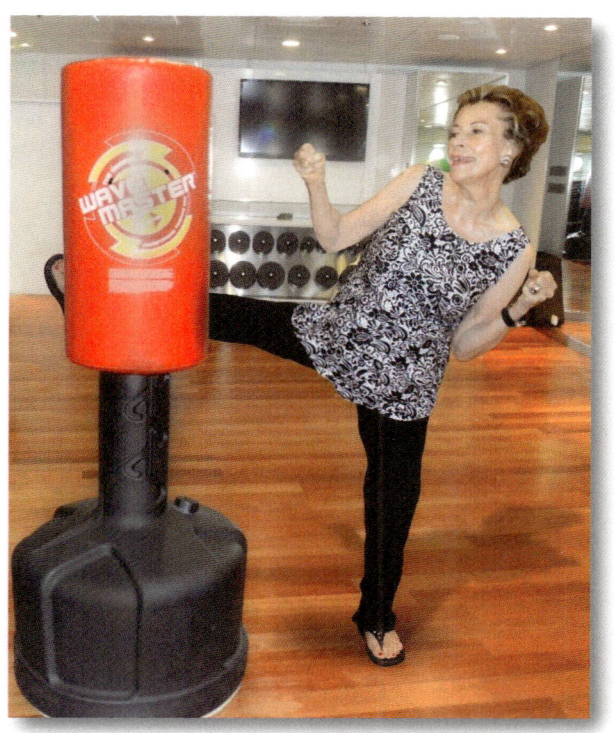

Exercise can and should be fun. If it is very hard work change it for something you can do and enjoy doing. Don't ruin the punching bag though!

Physiotherapy and exercising won't cure PD. The benefits may be short term at first and the exercises need to be continued. But exercise will slow the progress of PD symptoms.

It can have a positive impact on preventing or slowing freezing, reducing shuffling, and improving mobility. And you will almost certainly feel better.

Your posture will be helped and the stoop reduced or stabilized. And those painful joints, shoulders and knees are likely to stop aching, or not as much.

Doing it and being consistent with it is the key to success. Develop a regular schedule that you follow every day. Change it every month or six weeks so you do not get bored and also to make different muscle groups work.

Stretch every day and do it more than once. Help your posture straighten up and stretch against that friendly old wall.

Fun activities like Tai Chi and Pilates combine the friendship and chatter of the group with the real value of the exercises they offer. Spinning or marathon running might be a bit extreme, but do them anyway if you can and want to.

It is not only your body that needs exercising, your brain also needs stimulation, activity, excitement and interest.

Get involved in living, especially if you have let things slip a little. Revive that old hobby of photography, bird-watching, bridge or poker playing.

Walking on the beach, collecting shells or watching the tide take away the love letters in the sand, will keep you interested, improve your balance and increase your strength.

Stay living all and every part of your life.

Finally, flirting can still be fun and foolish!

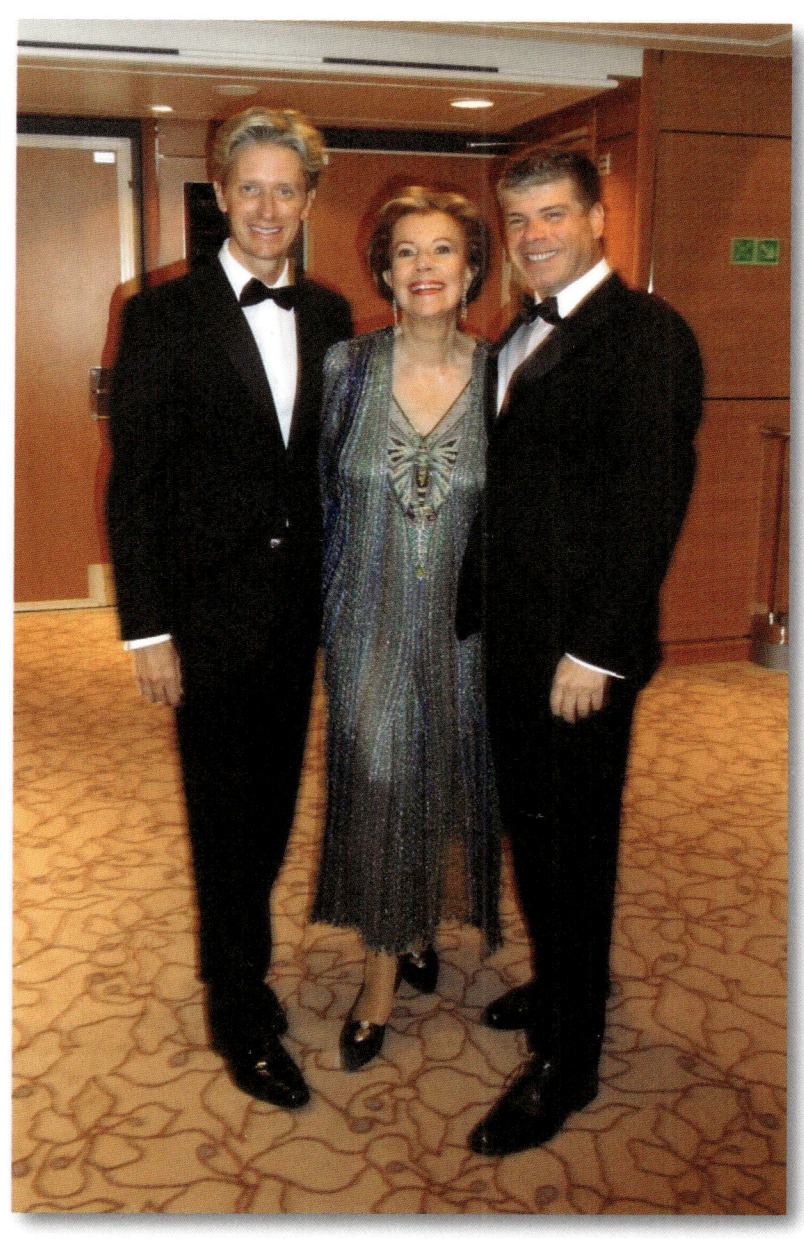

*They are all just good friends – of course!
Staying active in social life is very positive in living with PD.
Let it be the imposter while you live a real life.*

FROM NOW ONWARDS

So you know you have PD. It is in the early stages. There is a very long way to go before it gets to the advanced stages and you should be asking a lot of questions as the years go by.

Is PD preventable? Not yet is the truth.

No one has an answer and there is much debate. What causes the brain cells to stop producing dopamine is as yet unknown.

Several new drugs are undergoing testing. The role of vitamins, especially vitamin E, is being studied. Results are not all that great so far.

One day soon you might be using a pump that produces a levodopa gel right into your digestive system. It already exists in the USA and is very promising in creating less ups and downs and more stability. As ever it has side effects – including a not-so-social tendency to break wind at unwanted times.

A1A is not the old National Freeway. It is a new class of medicines that are rapidly coming through the testing pipeline. They are expected to improve your motor functions and also increase the amount of "ON" time.

If you have bad early morning "OFF" periods or if they are too slow in going away after your first dose, there is a way to speed things up. This is an injection of a drug called apomorphine that is available in most countries but it is not widely used.

So what else is new and coming up in the search for the treatment of PD's symptoms?

Well, back in ancient times the Greeks tricked the Trojans by building the famous Trojan Horse, filling it with Greeks and leaving the scene. The Trojans brought it into their citadel.

In the dead of night the Greeks left the horse and opened the gates and that was that for the Trojans.

There is a "Trojan Horse" being developed through gene research. It will try to insert a variety of different viruses into the cell's DNA through the genes.

The idea is that it will increase and control the dopamine production and thus reduce many of the motor symptoms. But it may have little effect on the other symptoms such as hallucination, depression and delusions. These will come later in new research.

Many other possible preventative treatments of symptoms are being researched. And so is the ultimate goal – a cure or a prevention.

It will take time, and one day it will be solved. When that is no one knows.

Can lost functions be restored?

It might be possible but much research and testing is still needed. Prevention of symptoms and delaying loss of function is still the best plan.

There is always a concern about the safety of treatments that could produce a worse outcome than the PD itself.

Be very wary of the Internet solutions to PD. Many of these are potentially harmful and misleading.

There is no danger in reading up on the latest discoveries or research. Being well informed is important. But don't try treating yourself with some of the untested and potentially dangerous "remedies" offered.

You will almost certainly be disappointed and they can very easily have serious outcomes.

PD is not to be played with. The specialist physicians and physios, the researchers and the dedicated medical people are working to help you and solve the riddles of PD. They are your real hope for the future.

Your best resources are your doctor, your physiotherapist, and yourself.

Can surgery help?

It might, but it has drawbacks – what else would you expect?

A part of the brain can be surgically stimulated and it seems to be benefiting advanced PD patients.

The surgeon operates on one side of the brain and the other side of the body responds. The patient will feel better and fitter.

It also works best with people under 65 and it has reduced slowness, the tremor, and rock and roll writhing. And that's good.

It does not seem to help much with balance and mobility. So that is not so good.

Surgery of this type is not for PD patients with dementia as it can actually worsen the problems.

But you do not have dementia or you would not be reading this.

Other surgical procedures involve planting electrodes in the brain.

Others try to stimulate the thalamus. All are in the beginning stages – but, once again, remember just how far medicine and surgery have come in the last ten years.

The sum of it all is that there is a ways to go before PD is fully understood, prevented and cured. But the work is intense, the knowledge base grows and sooner rather than later the breakthrough will come.

THE FUTURE AND YOU

The world goes on and you are well and truly in it. Plan to stay there and enjoy it to the fullest.

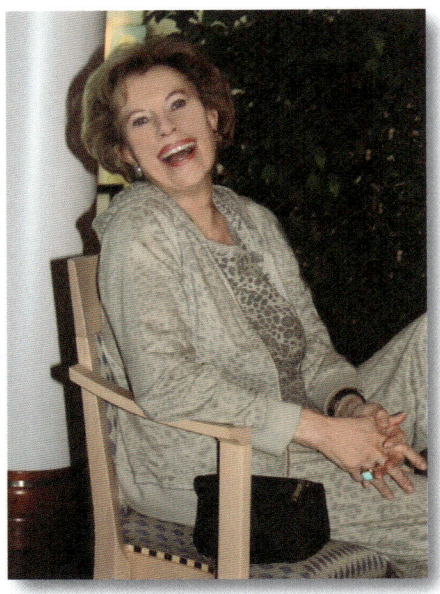

Laugh whenever and wherever you can.
Let it be a full throated belly buster and give it all you've got.
It's guaranteed to make you feel better and
it is a sure fire winner with your friends.
You have many years and many good things to do.

Medicine, physiotherapy, new research, new drugs and greater knowledge will all add to your quality of life as you live with PD. The researchers and the specialists may even find the answer everyone wants.

But the centrepiece of this true life reality show is not the PD. Nor will it be the professionals working to stem its progress and eliminate it.

The real star is, of course, you. You have it, live with it daily and have the power in you to take control of your life with PD.

Pauline was diagnosed in 2002. But she knows now that the symptoms were present some years before.

To date she has lived with diagnosed PD for 12 years and counting. She is now 84 years on from birth.

Look again at her in the photos.

They were taken by a friend with an iPad and others with ordinary digital cameras as she went through her daily, weekly and monthly life.

She suffers her bad moments with PD. She has her "ON" and "OFF" times, her symptoms are there, and are treated as we have talked about in prior pages.

So what is special about her?

Not a lot really that is anything more special than you or anyone else for that matter. Anything she has done to deal with PD you can do and so can almost everyone else, in one way or another.

It is all about attitude. Do you give up and let nature take its course? Do you blame the gods and devils for what has happened? Do you blame yourself?

Many people talk about fighting cancer or AIDS or PD. This is a start in the right direction for it means that they have decided to stay around.

You might prefer to see it a little differently, at least for now.

Think about living with PD while others fight it on your behalf. Don't waste your mental energy seeing it as a battle but as a problem you have that does not dominate every moment of your life.

You can control and counter it for many hours of every day, especially in the early years and you have a very long way to go before it becomes advanced.

If you have a partner, family, and or good friends they will love you all the greater if you continue to share your days with them, good and bad, but with a zest for being there and staying part of the great adventure of life.

And they can be a wonderful help to you in doing it.

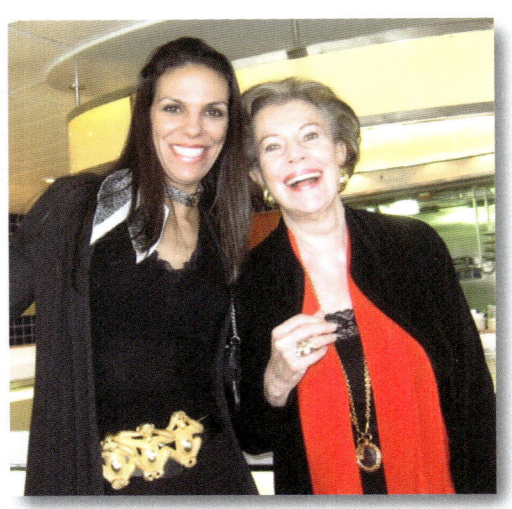

*This is Pauline's physiotherapist, Dr. Lisa Corsa who has helped her so much to live well with PD.
She and others like her are on the cutting edge of finding ways to control and stop the progress of PD.
Love your physio too!
Pauline has understood her lifestyle with PD and uses it to live each day to its utmost.*

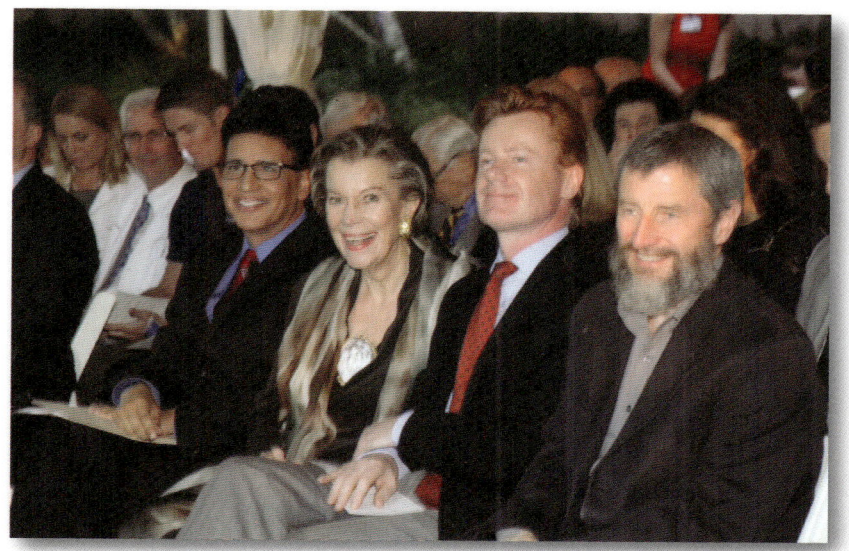

No matter where you are or where you go, take some friends along and make the most out of the day or night!.

Her best advice to you has already been presented in the photos and text in this book.

Her latest word on it might well be:

"It is your life to live, not Parkinson's"

COMMITMENT TO THE FUTURE

Pauline Braathen not only lives life with PD. She actively supports research and treatment.

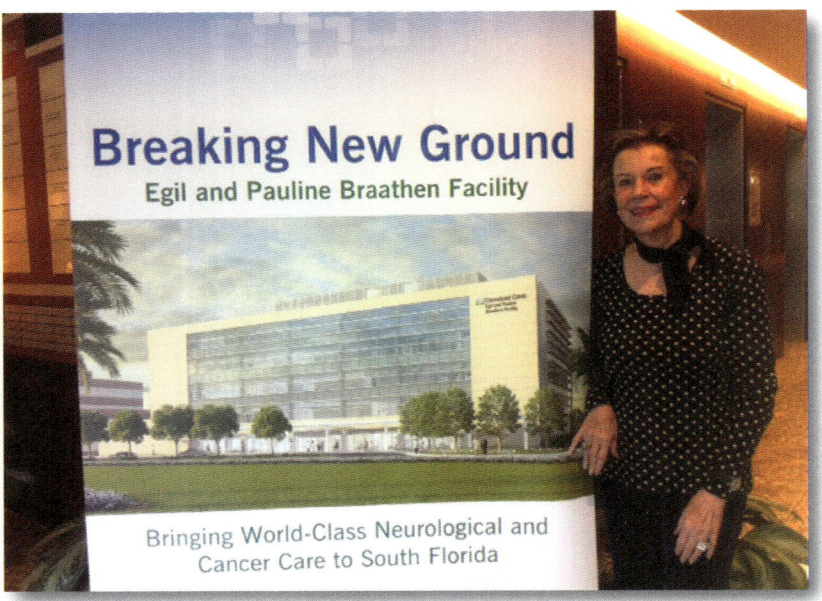

A new facility is being built at the Cleveland Clinic in Florida for PD patients. Perhaps it will one day help you to beat PD entirely or live with it in greater peace and comfort.

One day, perhaps soon, the applied research from facilities such as hers in the Cleveland Clinic will find the cause, cure and prevention of Parkinson's Disease.

In the meantime you and she have a life to enjoy and fulfill.

Live every moment of it.

ACKNOWLEDGEMENTS

This book could not and would not have been written without the essential contributions, guidance and support of the professionals acknowledged below.

Nestor Galvez-Jimenez MD MSc MS(HSA) FACP FANA FAHA

Chairman, Department of Neurology
Center Director, Pauline M. Braathen Neurosciences Center/Neurological Institute.
Chief, Movement Disorders Program, Cleveland Clinic Florida
Clinical Professor, Department of Neurology.
Herbert Wertheim College of Medicine Florida International University.

Dr. Galvez-Jimenez has provided invaluable and detailed medical information upon which the medical options described in the book are based. His research and applied neurology is outstanding in its field and he is one of the leading specialists worldwide in the search for prevention, treatment and cure of Parkinson's Disease.

Dr. Galvez-Jimenez is the author of several books and many articles in the field of neurology.

Without doubt, when Parkinson's Disease is finally conquered, as it will be, the work of Dr. Galvez-Jimenez will have been a vital and substantial contributor to that most welcome of outcomes.

Dr. Lisa Corsa DPT MSPT ATC LAT CPT LSVT-BIG

International Concierge Physiotherapy
Premier Therapy Solutions

Dr. Corsa is one of America's and the world's leading Physiotherapists. Her work in Theoretical and Applied Physiotherapy is cutting edge as are her treatment techniques and therapies.

The bulk and the best of the advice on physiotherapy applied to Parkinson's Disease in this book have been provided by Dr Corsa in excerpts from her manuscripts and directly to the writer.

Dr. Corsa's clinical expertise is second to none, not only in relation to PD but also in the wider field of physiotherapy in all its aspects.

A visit to her web site www.premierptsolutions.com is highly recommended.

Sharon Clark
Memoirist

The original concept of the book arose in discussions with Pauline and her biographer Sharon Clark. Since then it has been changed and expanded into the present text.

Throughout this process Sharon's writing and editing skills have added greatly to the development of the book.

WHO IS PAULINE?

A brilliant smile is the first thing you notice about Pauline Braathen. It's a reflection of her positive view of life, despite having PD.

One of Pauline's mottos is "Be grateful for what you have rather than complain about what you don't have."

An elegant English-woman, Pauline holds onto this maxim as she navigates through a remarkable life that has presented as many challenges as it has opportunities.

An attractive runway model in London at age eighteen, Pauline Heath quickly learned the business side of the trade and achieved the status of a top fashion buyer with offices in Bond Street, London.

On a 1963 holiday in the Canary Islands, Pauline was introduced to handsome Norwegian businessman Egil Braathen who swept her off her feet. She gave up her career and during their forty-six year marriage Pauline played a vital part in her husband's success.

As they shared extraordinary times from Oslo and London to Spain and the U.S., the years took their toll on Pauline's health. She survived numerous illnesses and operations, and in 2002 Pauline was diagnosed with Parkinson's Disease. She had experienced its symptoms for several years previously.

Through it all Pauline maintains a positive attitude and considers herself lucky to have found the right people to help her deal with Parkinson's. She doesn't talk about PD — she just wants to make life better for others with Parkinson's.

616.833 Bra
Braathen, Pauline,
PD, you and me.